Hormonal Control Systems

Supplement 1

Mathematical Biosciences

an international journal

Editor, Richard Bellman

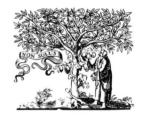

American Elsevier
Publishing Company, Inc.
New York, 1969

Hormonal Control Systems

Proceedings of the Symposium

held October 20-22, 1967

at Rancho Santa Fe, California

Edited by

EDWIN B. STEAR
Department of Engineering
University of California, Los Angeles

ARNOLD H. KADISII
Department of Electrical Engineering
California Institute of Technology, Pasadena

with the collaboration of

GEORGE BEKEY *and* CHARLES HAUN
University of Southern California, Los Angeles

CHARLES SAWYER
University of California, Los Angeles

R. SRIDHAR
California Institute of Technology, Pasadena

AMERICAN ELSEVIER PUBLISHING COMPANY, INC.
52 Vanderbilt Avenue, New York, N.Y. 10007

ELSEVIER PUBLISHING COMPANY, LTD.
Barking, Essex, England

ELSEVIER PUBLISHING COMPANY
335 Jan Van Galenstraat, P.O. Box 211
Amsterdam, The Netherlands

Standard Book Number 444-00064-X

Library of Congress Card Number 68-103147

Manufactured in the United States of America

PREFACE

In this volume the editors present the invited papers delivered at the first
of a planned series of inter-disciplinary conferences on Biological Control Systems
in Health and Disease. This first conference dealt with Hormonal Control Systems
and was held at Rancho Santa Fe, California on October 20-22, 1967. The conference
was organized to provide a forum for the meaningful exchange of ideas on an informal
as well as a formal basis between experienced researchers interested in the physiological and modeling aspects of hormonal regulation and control, and it was held
in an environment conducive to such an exchange of ideas. Participation in the conference was by invitation only and was intentionally limited to help promote the free
exchange of ideas between all participants. The appearance of this volume now makes
the material which was formally presented at the conference - and which formed the
basis for organized discussion sessions at the conference - available to everyone
interested in this fascinating area of inter-disciplinary research.

In order to help focus the discussion at the conference and yet not restrict
it too much, the organizing committee decided on a format which consisted of four
one-half day sessions, each of which was devoted to a particular hormonal system,
followed by a one-half day session devoted to two related aspects of biological control and regulation, each of which might form the basis of a future conference. The
four hormonal systems covered were (1) adrenal cortical function, (2) glucose and
metabolic fuel homeostasis, (3) thyroid function, and (4) gonadal function. In
each of these four areas, leading researchers were invited to present a paper cov-
ering the known physiology of the system which is pertinent to hormonal regulation
and control and a paper devoted to the control and modeling aspects of the system.
The two related aspects covered were brain-endocrine relationships and biological
control at the molecular level with an invited paper on each of these subjects being
presented by internationally known researchers. These ten papers form the content
of this volume.

A unique feature of this conference, as reflected in the invited papers presented and in the invited conference participants, was that it brought together approximately equal numbers of experienced researchers who were medicine and/or biology oriented and experienced researchers who were engineering, mathematics, and/or physics oriented for a truly inter-disciplinary conference. We feel that our goal of encouraging greater mutual interaction between these somewhat diverse groups of researchers was achieved in great measure. This was attested to by the almost unanimous impression of the participants in the conference, each of whom was invited because of his interest and demonstrated accomplishment in the general area of biological control and regulation. We have been fortunate indeed in our contributors whose scholarship, critique, and appraisal are evident. It is hoped that others in this field or in cognate fields will derive some real benefit from this unique work.

We wish to acknowledge the collaboration of our fellow members of the organizing committee for the conference. The success of the conference was due in great measure to their efforts. They were Drs. George Bekey and Charles Haun of the University of Southern California, Dr. Charles Sawyer of the University of California, Los Angeles, and Dr. R. Sridhar of the California Institute of Technology. In addition, we wish to acknowledge the substantial support of Dr. Merle Andrew, Dr. Harvey Savely, and Dr. Allen Dayton of the Air Force Office of Scientific Research without which the conference could not have been held.

We also wish to acknowledge the informal contributions of Dr. Dinesh Sharma to the organization of the conference in its very early formative stages and his proofreading of a large segment of the final manuscript. Finally, we wish to thank Mrs. Betty Leventhal for her excellent handling of the administrative aspects of the conference and Miss Lois Howard for her excellent job of typing the final manuscript in camera ready copy under trying circumstances.

The conference was organized under the sponsorship of the University of California, Los Angeles, The California Institute of Technology, The University of Southern California, The Metabolic Dynamics Foundation, Inc., and the Directorate of Mathematical Sciences and the Directorate of Life Sciences of the Air Force Office of Scientific Research. The administrative aspects of the conference were very ably handled by the Engineering Extension Office of the Department of Engineering, University of California, Los Angeles and financial support of the conference was provided by the Applied Mathematics Division of the Directorate of Mathematical Sciences and by The Directorate of Life Sciences, Air Force Office of Scientific Research under AFOSR Grant No. AFOSR-68-1429.

April 1969   Edwin Stear, Ph.D.
                                             University of California, Los Angeles

                                             Arnold Kadish, M.D.
                                             California Institute of Technology

CONTENTS

CONTRIBUTORS

R.D. BRENNAN
IBM Scientific Center
Palo Alto, California

(pp. 20-87)

K. BROWN-GRANT
Department of Human Anatomy
University of Oxford
Oxford, England

(pp. 150-160)

G.F. CAHILL, JR.
Department of Medicine
Elliott P. Joslin Research Laboratory
Harvard Medical School and
Peter Bent Brigham Hospital and the
Diabetes Foundation, Inc.,
Boston, Massachusetts

(pp. 88-114)

W.P. CHARETTE
Department of Electrical Engineering
California Institute of Technology
Pasadena, California

(pp. 115-149)

D.B. CRIGHTON
Department of Physiology
University of Texas Southwestern
  Medical School
Dallas, Texas

(pp. 193-228)

A.P.S DHARIWAL
Department of Physiology
University of Texas Southwestern
  Medical School
Dallas, Texas

(pp. 193-228)

JOSEPH J. DISTEFANO III
Department of Engineering
University of California, Los Angeles
Los Angeles, California

(pp. 161-192)

RENATO DULBECCO
The Salk Institute for Biological Studies
La Jolla, California

(pp. 280-288)

WILLIAM F. GANONG
School of Medicine
San Francisco Medical Center
University of California
San Francisco, California

(pp. 256-279)

A.H. KADISH
Department of Electrical Engineering
California Institute of Technology
Pasadena, California

(pp. 115-149)

GRANT W. LIDDLE
Department of Medicine
Vanderbilt University School of Medicine
Nashville, Tennessee

(pp. 1-19)

S.M. McCANN
Department of Physiology
University of Texas Southwestern
  Medical School
Dallas, Texas

(pp. 193-228)

NEENA B. SCHWARTZ
College of Medicine
University of Illinois
Chicago, Illinois

(pp. 229-255)

J.S. SOELDNER
Department of Medicine
Elliott P. Joslin Research Laboratory
Harvard Medical School and
Peter Bent Brigham Hospital and the
Diabetes Foundation, Inc.,
Boston, Massachusetts

(pp. 88-114)

R. SRIDHAR
Department of Electrical Engineering
California Institute of Technology
Pasadena, California

(pp. 115-149)

EDWIN B. STEAR
Department of Engineering
University of California, Los Angeles
Los Angeles, California

(pp. 161-192)

S. WATANABE
Department of Physiology
University of Texas Southwestern
  Medical School
Dallas, Texas

(pp. 193-228)

J.T. WATSON
Department of Physiology
University of Texas Southwestern
  Medical School
Dallas, Texas

(pp. 193-228)

F.E. YATES
Department of Physiology
Stanford University
Stanford, California

(pp. 20-87)

I. PHYSIOLOGICAL REVIEW OF ADRENOCORTICAL FUNCTION

GRANT W. LIDDLE
Department of Medicine, Vanderbilt University School of Medicine, Nashville, Tennessee

---

INTRODUCTION

It is the purpose of this paper to describe the salient facts of adrenocortical physiology that must be taken into consideration in any adequate attempt to construct on analogous physicomathematical model. First, some of the intra-adrenal factors determining the rate of corticosteroidogenesis will be mentioned. Then, some of the factors influencing the secretion of ACTH[**] will be described. Finally, some of the aberrations of pituitary-adrenal function encountered in clinical medicine will be characterized.

For the sake of brevity, only the major glucocorticoids will be considered: cortisol in man and corticosterone in the rat. Aldosterone, the principal mineralocorticoid, is regulated by a different mechanism and need not be considered here. Although I shall not dwell on the subject, it must be mentioned that in human plasma there is a globulin with high affinity for cortisol, designated by various investigators as "transcortin" or "cortisol binding globulin." The quantity of this protein in the plasma increases during pregnancy and during treatment with estrogens. It is virtually absent in certain families. The reversible binding of cortisol to transcortin and ot other plasma proteins does not modify the regulation of cortisol secretion or metabolism in any major way and, furthermore, can readily be provided for by modeling experts. It must also be pointed out (and again the modeling experts

---

*Original data reported in this paper were obtained in studies supported in part by grants-in-aid from the National Institutes of Health, USPHS 5 R01 AM 05318, 5 T01 AM 05092, 4 K6 AM 3782, and 8 M01 FR 95.

** The following abbreviations will be employed: "ACTH" = adrenocorticotropic hormone; 17-OHCS=17-hydroxycorticosteroids (cortisol and substance S and their metabolites).

GRANT W. LIDDLE

will have no difficulty with this) that cortisol is metabolized by the liver to
biologically inactive products. In normal subjects, cortisol is removed from the
circulation with a "half-time" of a little more than one hour. The removal of cortisol from the circulation is accelerated in hyperthyroidism and is retarded in hypothyroidism and in hepatic insufficiency.

A dominant theme throughout the paper will be the functional interdependence of
the pituitary and adrenal glands. The normal adrenal secretes appreciable quantities
of corticosteroids only in response to ACTH, and corticosteroids in turn suppress the
secretion of ACTH. Pituitary-adrenal physiology is by no means that simple, however.
There are many intra-adrenal factors that help to determine the effectiveness of ACTH
in stimulating corticosteroid secretion and many factors other than corticosteroids
that help to determine the rate of secretion of ACTH by the pituitary.

INTRA-ADRENAL DETERMINANTS OF CORTICOSTEROID SECRETION AND THE MECHANISM OF ACTION
OF ACTH

Some of the major steps in the corticosteroid biosynthetic pathway are shown in
Figure 1. The adrenal cortex is capable of utilizing acetate to synthesize cholesterol, which in turn serves as a precursor for corticosteroids [20]. Each of the
reactions is catalyzed by one or more enzyme systems; therefore, each step is potentially rate-limiting. The argument that the conversion of cholesterol to Δ^5-preg-
nenolone is regulated by ACTH and that this is normally the rate-limiting [46] step
in corticosteroid biosynthesis runs as follows. Even in the absence of ACTH there
is a large amount of cholesterol in the adrenal; therefore, the pre-cholesterol
steps in corticosteroid biosynthesis are not ordinarily rate-limiting. Even in the
absence of ACTH the (rat) adrenal is capable of effecting the rapid conversion of
Δ^5-pregnenolone to corticosterone [14]; therefore, the post-pregnenolone steps in
corticosteroid biosynthesis are not ordinarily rate-limiting. By exclusion, therefore, the failure of the adrenal to carry out the synthesis of corticosteroids in
the absence of ACTH must be due to its limited capacity to convert cholesterol to
Δ^5-pregnenolone. This capacity is greatly increased by the action of ACTH, for over
a considerable dose-response range the rate of conversion of cholesterol to corticosteroids is directly proportional to the quantity of ACTH in contact with adrenal
cells.

The dynamics of adrenocortical activation in response to ACTH have been elegantly described by Urquhart in recent studies of the perfused dog adrenal [52]. An
account of this work will be found elsewhere in this symposium and so will not be
dealt with here. In general, what Urquhart has found in the perfused dog adrenal

is consistent with what has been learned using less direct methods in intact man [11] and rat [30]. In brief, ACTH has no appreciable effect on corticosterone or cortisol secretion for the first 3 or 4 minutes after it is injected. There is then a sharp rise in corticosteroid secretion, the amplitude and duration of which are both functions of the dose of ACTH [30]. Near maximum secretory responses are a-chieved with plasma ACTH concentrations of 3 milli-units (mU) per 100 ml or greater in man [38]. In the rat, a maximum 10 minute response is elicited by the instantane-ous intravenous injection of 1 mU or more into the whole animal [30]. ACTH disappears from the circulation with a half-time of several minutes, and corticosteroid secretion falls to negligible levels within several minutes after the last of the ACTH disap-pears from the circulation. On the other hand, corticosteroid secretion continues as long as ACTH persists in the circulation, and the phenomenon of "adrenal exhaustion," though written about in the early days of experimental adrenal physiology, has never been documented by adequate methods.

The biochemical events leading to the acute rise in corticosteroid secretion that occurs after the injection of ACTH have been extensively investigated, but they are still incompletely understood. These will be summarized first, and then some longer-term effects of ACTH on adrenocortical capacity to produce corticosteroids will be described.

Within 1 minute after ACTH reaches the adrenal, and well ahead of any appreciable increase in corticosteroid secretion, there is a sharp increase in the intracellular concentration of cyclic AMP (3',5'-adenosine monophosphate) [17]. The degree of rise in cyclic AMP is a function of the dose of ACTH. Cyclic AMP remains elevated as long as ACTH is present; but after ACTH is removed from the system, adrenal cyclic AMP quickly returns to basal levels. The rise and fall in adrenal cyclic AMP is followed closely by a rise and fall in corticosteroid secretion. In the absence of ACTH, ex-ogenous cyclic AMP is capable of stimulating corticosteroid secretion in much the same way as does ACTH itself [22]. Because ACTH stimulates the formation of cyclic AMP and because cyclic AMP produces effects similar to those of ACTH, it is thought that cyclic AMP is the intracellular mediator of the steroidogenic action of ACTH. It has been shown that the acute action of both agents is to stimulate the conver-sion of cholesterol to Δ^5-pregnenolone. It is thought that this conversion is me-diated by a labile protein, since it is blocked by a variety of inhibitors of pro-tein synthesis [9, 10, 14, 17]. Such inhibitors do not interfere with the formation of cyclic AMP, so that, when one gives ACTH in the presence of an inhibitor of pro-tein synthesis, cyclic AMP increases but corticosteroid secretion does not [17].

GRANT W. LIDDLE

It is well-known that over a finite period of time the capacity of the adrenal to respond to ACTH is limited; there is a point beyond which increments in ACTH concentration do not evoke further increases in corticosteroid secretion [30]. This is also true when cyclic AMP is used as the stimulator of steroidogenesis [17]. Furthermore, it has been shown that the addition of exogenous cyclic AMP does not increase the steroidogenic activity of adrenal tissue that is already "maximally" stimulated by ACTH [24]. This observation is consistent with the view that ACTH and cyclic AMP act through the same mechanism to stimulate steroidogenesis and the view that the effect of ACTH is mediated by cyclic AMP.

The studies of Grahame-Smith and co-workers [17] indicate that the adrenal response to ACTH is limited not by the number of receptor sites for ACTH nor by the amount of cyclic AMP that can be formed in response to ACTH but, rather, by some step subsequent to cyclic AMP formation. These investigators found that "small" doses of ACTH stimulated more-or-less proportional increases in cyclic AMP formation and corticosteroid secretion up to the point where maximal steroidogenesis was achieved. By increasing the dose of ACTH further, it was possible to bring about a further 80-fold increase in cyclic AMP formation without further increases in steroidogenesis.

It has been shown that the addition of NADPH to the adrenal in vitro stimulates corticosteroid synthesis [18]. Whether the formation of NADPH is itself stimulated by ACTH and cyclic AMP is uncertain. Adrenal concentrations of NADPH have not been shown to rise in response to steroidogenic doses of ACTH. It is theoretically possible, however, that the concentration of NADPH at some critical site in the adrenocortical cell might be increased as a result of the action of ACTH. At least two processes through which ACTH might stimulate the formation of NADPH have been proposed. Haynes and co-workers [19] have shown that under certain circumstances, ACTH and cyclic AMP bring about an increase in adrenal phosphorylase. Phosphorylase catalyzes the breakdown of glycogen to form glucose-1-phosphate, which is rapidly converted to glucose-6-phosphate. The metabolism of glucose-6-phosphate by a dehydrogenase in the presence of NADP leads to the generation of NADPH. According to an alternative theory proposed by McKerns [36], ACTH activates glucose-6-phosphate dehydrogenase, thus promoting the reduction of NADP to NADPH, which in turn stimulates steroidogenesis. Despite the fact that the subject has been vigorously and ingeniously investigated, there is still no generally accepted, totally integrated concept of the mechanism through which ACTH stimulates the conversion of cholesterol to Δ^5-pregnenolone and thus regulates the rate of steroidogenesis [21].

The fact that ACTH has a regulatory effect on the rate-limiting step of corticosteroid synthesis does not mean that the role of ACTH is restricted to this action alone. Ney and co-workers [39] have adduced evidence that ACTH promotes the synthesis of the relatively stable adrenal proteins that are involved in the late steps of steroidogenesis; i.e., the enzyme systems that convert Δ^5-pregnenolone to corticosterone. The biologic importance of this action of ACTH could be that of maintaining the efficiency of the later steps of the steroidogenic pathway so that they can always accommodate the quantity of Δ^5-pregnenolone formed as a result of the acute action of ACTH. Furthermore, recent studies by Dexter and co-workers [4] have shown that ACTH has a direct stimulatory effect on cholesterol anabolism by the adrenal cortex. This action of ACTH could be of biologic importance in assuring the continuing availability of cholesterol to serve as a steroid precursor. Were it not for the subtle long-term trophic effects of ACTH on the early and late steps of the steroidogenic pathway, circumstances might develop in which these steps (rather than the acutely activated cholesterol-to-Δ^5-pregnenolone step) would be rate-limiting.

The capacity of the adrenal to secrete corticosteroids in response to ACTH at any one moment is a function of its trophic history. If the adrenal is atrophic due to chronic lack of ACTH, the acute response to a pulse of ACTH is small. If the adrenal is hyperplastic due to a chronic excess of ACTH, the steroidogenic capacity is large [48]. A trophic influence of ACTH is apparent even within a few hours. In the rat, within 24 hours after hypophysectomy, there is a four-fold decrease in steroidogenic response to a pulse of ACTH [30]. In man, continuous suppression of endogenous ACTH reduces the responsiveness of the adrenal to 50% of its original level within a period of 2 days, if responsiveness is tested by the intravenous infusion of standard doses of exogenous ACTH. In contrast, repetitive treatment with ACTH, infused intravenously for several hours a day on several successive days, results in progressive enhancement of the steroidogenic response [26].

The priming influence of ACTH in preparing the adrenal gland to respond to subsequent exposure to ACTH is apparent in many ways. For example, there is normally a diurnal rhythm in ACTH secretion, with a crest during the morning and a trough in the evening [5, 11, 42, 44, 45], and this fact serves to explain why the adrenal is more responsive to a test dose of ACTH given late in the morning than it is to a similar dose given late in the evening [41, 44, 45]. As has been pointed out by Nugent and co-workers [41], patients with Cushing's disease lack a diurnal rhythm in adrenal responsiveness, and this can be explained by their lack of a normal diurnal rhythm in ACTH secretion.

GRANT W. LIDDLE

REGULATION OF ACTH SECRETION

There are three known factors that influence ACTH secretion in man. First is the influence of sleep-wake habits, making for a diurnal rhythm in ACTH secretion. Second is the influence of stress. A variety of noxious stimuli (major injuries, infections, hypoglycemia, etc.) bring about increased secretion of ACTH. It need not be assumed that all act through a common mechanism. Third is the influence of cortisol-like steroids. To some extent the pituitary-adrenal system behaves like a negative feedback mechanism: the higher the level of cortisol, the greater is the restraint on ACTH secretion and, therefore, the less stimulation of further cortisol secretion. The operation of each of these three influences on ACTH secretion under experimental and clinical conditions will be described. Then their interactions, when they are set in opposition to each other, will be considered.

1. Diurnal Rhythmicity in ACTH Secretion [40]. In normal subjects who conform to a regular sleep-wake schedule, ACTH secretion rises during sleep, reaching a peak at about the time of awakening. It then falls irregularly during the waking day, reaching a minimum at about the beginning of the next sleep period. Since most people are in the habit of sleeping at night and being awake during the day, the usual ACTH-cortisol secretory pattern is characterized by high values in the morning and low values in the evening. It has been shown that this pattern is not well- established during the first few months of life [12]. Furthermore, it is possible to alter the pattern experimentally by revising an individual's sleep-wake habits [42, 44]. For example, if a normal subject habitually sleeps 4 hours and is then awake for 8 hours so that he has two sleep-wake cycles per 24 hours, his pituitary-adrenal activity will, after several days, conform to this sleep-awake schedule with two sleep-correlated cycles per day [33].

Precisely how the pituitary-adrenal rhythm becomes entrained to follow one's sleep-wake schedule is unknown. The immediate act of sleeping or waking is not the direct determinant of pituitary-adrenal activity, however, for radical alteration of the habitual sleep-wake schedule for a single day does not immediately alter the established pituitary-adrenal rhythm [42]. In the absence of fundamental understanding of the mechanism involved, it is convenient to resort to the superficial explanation that the rise in ACTH secretion that occurs prior to awakening each day is a conditioned response representing somehow the subconscious anticipation of awakening.

A diurnal rhythm is characteristic not only of normal subjects but also of most patients. Notable exceptions occur in patients who are obviously stressed [44], in certain patients with central nervous system lesions (especially pretectal in location) [25], and in patients with Cushing's syndrome [6,7,34].

2. <u>Stress</u>. For over 20 years it has been known that a variety of severe stresses will bring about increased pituitary-adrenal activity. Although the unifying concept "stress" has has a certain usefulness, it has also been deceptive. The term "stress" means many things to many people. Not all insults to the organism, even life-threatening insults, stimulate ACTH secretion. Furthermore, the various noxious stimuli that do stimulate ACTH secretion might or might not exert their effects through a common mechanism. For example, in patients with Cushing's disease, the pituitary-adrenal response to insulin-induced hypoglycemia is impaired even though the response to laparotomy is intact. In dogs, it has been shown that a pituitary-adrenal response to hypoglycemia ceases after a time despite persistence of the hypoglycemia; the hypoglycemia-unresponsive pituitary can then be induced to secrete ACTH by addition of a noxious stimulus of another modality [55].

In endocrinologically normal human subjects, pituitary-adrenal responses to the following stimuli have been characterized.

Λ. <u>Laparotomy</u>. The following statements about the pituitary-adrenal response to the stress of laparotomy are derived largely from the studies of Estep and co-workers [8]. Twenty women studied during pelvic laparotomy were found to have increases in plasma ACTH from pre-operative values of 0.1 to 0.4 mU per 100 ml to values of 0.4 to 1.5 mU per 100 ml. Plasma 17-hydroxycorticosteroids (17-OHCS) rose from pre-operative values of 6 to 22 µg per 100 ml to values of 15 to 45 µg per 100 ml and remained elevated for several hours following completion of the operation. Urinary 17-OHCS increased from pre-operative values of 3 to 9 mg per day to values of 8 to 20 mg on the day of the operation.

Although the pituitary-adrenal responses to laparotomy were distinct in every case, the plasma ACTH concentrations and the plasma and urinary 17-OHCS values were not as high as those usually observed when normal subjects are given infusions of ACTH at rates in excess of 1 unit per hour. In other words, in response to laparotomy, the pituitary usually does not secrete enough ACTH to elicit a maximal adrenal secretory response.

Somewhat less formidable surgical operations, such as hemorrhoidectomy or repair of an incisional hernia, are frequently unassociated with an obvious increase in pituitary-adrenal activity.

GRANT W. LIDDLE

B. Pyrogens. The injection of pyrogenic doses of certain bacterial poly-
saccharide complexes results in an increase in plasma 17-OHCS in subjects
with intact pituitaries and responsive adrenals. The response is eva-
nescent, and 17-OHCS return to normal within a few hours. The 17-OHCS response is mediated by a transient increase in ACTH secretion [50]. Usually
the response is not of sufficient duration to result in an obvious increase in the 24-hour excretion of 17-OHCS in the urine.

C. Hypoglycemia. The induction of acute hypoglycemia with insulin results in
a brisk increase in plasma 17-OHCS with a subsequent return to control values even though the hypoglycemia is maintained [55]. The normal 17-OHCS
response is frequently absent in patients with hypothalamic lesions and,
curiously, in patients with Cushing's syndrome.

D. Electroshock. Passage of a current of electricity through the head, in
the manner employed in the treatment of psychiatric disorders, results in
a distinct increase in plasma 17-OHCS [30].

Other noxious stimuli [13] such as histamine injections, burns, electrical stimulation of the sciatic nerve, and other anesthesia have been
found to stimulate ACTH secretion in animals, and psychological trauma
[35] associated with extreme fear or anger has been found to stimulate a
rise in plasma 17-OHCS in man, presumably through stimulation of ACTH
secretion.

3. Negative Feedback Regulation by Corticosteroids. Cortisol is the one product of the human adrenal that is both potent enough and abundant enough to regulate
the secretion of ACTH by the pituitary. In normal physiology, cortisol is secreted
only in response to ACTH, and the amount of ACTH secreted by the pituitary is an
inverse function of the level of cortisol. The higher the level of cortisol, the
greater is its restraining influence on ACTH secretion; the lower the level of cortisol, the less the restraint on ACTH secretion. In this fashion ACTH and cortisol
levels tend to be self-regulating and normally remain within rather narrow limits.

In patients with cortisol-secreting adrenal neoplasms and in patients receiving
supraphysiologic doses of exogenous cortisol, the production of ACTH is suppressed
[15,23,43] so that ACTH secretion falls to negligible quantities, and the concentration of ACTH in the pituitary gradually decreases. In contrast, in patients
whose adrenocortical function is compromised [16,51] as a consequence of some de-
structive process (surgery, tuberculosis, autoimmune atrophy, etc.) or as a consequence of enzyme inhibition (genetic or pharmacologic), there occurs a compensatory
increase in pituitary production of ACTH. This compensatory increase can be quickly

curtailed by the administration of physiologic quantities of cortisol.

In recent years several pharmacologic agents have been developed which inhibit various steps in the corticosteroid biosynthetic pathway. A decrease in corticosterone secretion in the rat or cortisol secretion in man calls forth a compensatory increase in ACTH secretion, so that partial inhibition of steroid biosynthesis might be overridden by increased activity of the ACTH-responsive steps in the pathway. The steroid intermediate occurring just prior to the inhibited step is secreted in increased quantities. The most intensively studied adrenal inhibitor is metyrapone [27, 28]. This agent inhibits 11β-hydroxylation, leading to a decrease in cortisol secretion and the appearance in the plasma of the immediate precursor of cortisol, 11-deoxycortisol, otherwise known as Reichstein's substance S. As a consequence of decreased cortisol secretion, there is a compensatory increase in ACTH secretion. The metyrapone inhibited adrenal responds to an increase in plasma ACTH by secreting more substance S and more cortisol until cortisol levels are restored to normal. Normalization of cortisol is thus achieved only at the cost of increased production of ACTH and increased production of cortisol precursors. Substance S and its metabolites are readily measurable in biologic fluids as 17-OHCS. In normal subjects, therefore, metyrapone induces a rise in total blood and urinary 17-OHCS consisting of both cortisol and "S" and their metabolites. Since this response to metyrapone is dependent upon both a rise in ACTH secretion and an increase in adrenal activity in response to the rise in ACTH, it affords a means of testing the reserve capacity of the pituitary-adrenal system. If a patient fails to respond to metyrapone with an increase in 17-OHCS, it can be assumed either that there was no increase in his ACTH secretion or that his adrenals were unresponsive to augmented ACTH secretion. If his adrenals are responsive to exogenous ACTH, it may be assumed that his failure to respond to metyrapone with an increase in 17-OHCS was attributable to a failure of the pituitary to secrete ACTH rather than a failure of the adrenals to respond to ACTH. In combination with a standard ACTH test, then, metyrapone can be used in the assessment of "pituitary ACTH reserve."

4. Interactions of Various Determinants of ACTH Secretion. The identification of 3 distinct determinants of ACTH secretion has made it possible to inquire which of any pair of these determinants would dominate pituitary regulation if they were set in opposition to each other. The following studies have attempted to explore this question.

GRANT W. LIDDLE

A. <u>Stress vs. Diurnal Rhythm.</u> Although nonstressed subjects usually show decreasing plasma 17-OHCS concentrations during the course of the waking day, this trend is sharply reversed if a laparotomy is performed. The "stress" results in an abrupt rise in ACTH secretion, which results in increases in plasma and urinary 17-OHCS.

B. <u>Stress vs. Negative Feedback.</u> Although slightly supraphysiologic quantities of cortisol suppress ACTH secretion in nonstressed subjects, this so-called negative feedback mechanism fails to control ACTH secretion during certain major stresses. For example, the usual response to pelvic laparotomy includes elevation of plasma 17-OHCS to about 30 to 50 µg per 100 ml. One might think that this degree of elevation of plasma 17-OHCS would restrain the secretion of ACTH by the pituitary. It has been shown, however, that plasma ACTH concentrations become elevated during laparotomy even if cortisol is infused in quantities sufficient to maintain a plasma 17-OHCS concentration of 100 to 500 µg per 100 ml. Thus, severe stress provides a stimulus to ACTH secretion that overrides the "negative-feed-back" and "diurnal rhythm" influences on pituitary function [8].

C. <u>Diurnal Rhythm vs. Negative Feedback.</u> The normal pituitary responds to a deficiency of cortisol with a compensatory increase in ACTH secretion. Plasma ACTH concentrations may rise to 10 to 100 times normal. Even in the presence of a continuous deficiency of cortisol, however, the pituitary shows a diurnal variation in ACTH secretion. Thus, in addisonian patients maintained on suboptimal cortisol therapy given in constant dosage (every 2 hours "around the clock") plasma ACTH concentrations are high in the morning but fall to relatively low values in the evening [16]. It would appear, therefore, that the influence of one's habitual sleep schedule on ACTH secretion must be very powerful if it can bring about a decrease in the secretion of this hormone even in the presence of continuous cortisol deficiency.

CLINICAL ABERRATIONS OF PITUITARY-ADRENAL FUNCTION

There are six clinical disorders that I should like to characterize biologically in the hope that the characterizations might provide grist for the mills of the physicomathematical modelers.

1.   Addison's disease occurs as a consequence of virtually total destruction of the adrenal cortices. Cortisol secretion falls. ACTH secretion rises [51] to levels sufficient to induce maximal stimulation of any surviving adrenocortical remnants. Diurnal rhythmicity of ACTH secretion is retained [16] and so is pituitary responsiveness to stress [47]. Treatment with physiologic doses of cortisol results in a decrease in ACTH to normal [2].

2.   Congenital adrenal hyperplasia occurs as a consequence of an inherited defect in some specific step in the corticosteroid biosynthetic pathway [3]. In some cases cortisol secretion is subnormal, but in other "well-compensated" cases cortisol secretion is normal. ACTH secretion is greater than normal [49]. There is increased secretion of the steroid intermediate that occurs just prior to the defective step in the biosynthetic pathway leading to cortisol synthesis. In the "compensated" cases, treatment with metyrapone leads to a further increase in ACTH secretion by the pituitary and substance S secretion by the adrenal cortex [28]. Treatment with physiologic doses of cortisol results in a reduction of ACTH to normal, and the secretion of precursor steroids also falls to normal [1,53].

3.   Cushing's disease occurs as a consequence of excessive secretion of ACTH by the pituitary. For a given rate of cortisol secretion (or administration), the patient with Cushing's disease secretes more ACTH than would a normal nonstressed individual. Cortisol secretion is greater than normal, and diurnal rhythmicity in in pituitary-adrenal function is usually lost [6,7,34]. The pituitary retains it responsiveness to stress, and the adrenal glands respond vigorously to standard test doses of exogenous ACTH [30]. In response to metyrapone-induced impairment of cortisol synthesis, there is a further increase in ACTH secretion by the pituitary and in 17-OHCS secretion by the adrenals [28]. It is only by administering corticosteroids in distinctly supraphysiologic doses that one can curtail ACTH production to the point that the adrenal glands cease to secrete supernormal quantities of cortisol [29]. If, by subtotal adrenalectomy, one reduces cortisol secretion to normal, ACTH secretion increases even further [54].

The facts that large doses of corticosteroids can suppress ACTH secretion and that ACTH secretion increases both in response to metyrapone and in response to normalization of cortisol secretion by means of subtotal adrenalectomy all indicate that a negative feedback mechanism of some sort is still operative in governing the secretion of ACTH in Cushing's disease. However, there are several reasons for believing that this negative feedback mechanism works with rather poor precision. For example, it often takes much more exogenous corticosteroid to suppress pituitary-

GRANT W. LIDDLE

adrenal function in the patient with Cushing's disease than one would predict on the basis of the cortisol secretion rate.

Still another indication that the negative feedback mechanism is cumbersome in Cushing's disease is illustrated in Figure 2. In normal subjects the intravenous infusion of 50 units of ACTH over an 8-hour period is accompanied by a rise in plasma and urinary 17-OHCS, which then return to control values within a few hours after the infusion of ACTH is terminated. In contrast, in the patient with Cushing's disease, the 17-OHCS often do not return to pre-infusion values but remain elevated for several days following a standard infusion of exogenous ACTH.

The abnormality of pituitary-adrenal function illustrated in Figure 2 can be explained in the following way. First, it can be assumed that an infusion of exogenous ACTH increases the subsequent sensitivity of the adrenals to endogenous ACTH, both in normal subjects and in patients with Cushing's disease. Second, it can be assumed that the normal pituitary secretes only that amount of ACTH that is appropriate to bring cortisol secretion to normal. Therefore, if the adrenals are usually responsive to ACTH following the infusion of exogenous ACTH, the secretion of endogenous ACTH should be appropriately reduced so that the rate of production of cortisol should be the same as prior to treatment. Third, it is postulated that in Cushing's disease the secretion of ACTH by the pituitary is not precisely adjusted to the cortisol level. During the post-infusion period, ACTH continues to be secreted and acts on adrenals that have had their responsiveness enhanced by the recent infusion of exogenous ACTH. The adrenal response does not return to pre-infusion levels until the effect of the infusion in enhancing adrenal responsiveness has been dissipated, a process that requires several days for completion. An analogous phenomenon is also observed in the "ectopic ACTH syndrome," a condition in which "negative feedback" control of ACTH secretion is not merely cumberson but non-existent (vide infra).

4.   The "ectopic ACTH syndrome" [30,31,32,37] occurs as a consequence of autonomous elaboration of ACTH by a nonpituitary neoplasm. Plasma ACTH levels are high, and cortisol is excessively secreted, often to an extreme degree. Pituitary ACTH content decreases. The production of ectopic ACTH does not appear to be regulated by any of the factors that normally control the secretion of ACTH by the pituitary. There is no apparent diurnal rhythm in the secretion of ectopic ACTH. Exogenous corticosteroids, even in very large doses are generally ineffective in suppressing 17-OHCS, and this is of diagnostic value in separating patients with hypercortisolism due to ectopic ACTH from those with hypercortisolism due to pituitary ACTH (Cushing's disease).

The response to metyrapone depends upon the severity of the cortisol excess.

Patients with only modest elevations of cortisol secretion usually respond to metyrapone with further increases in total 17-OHCS secretion. Those with extreme elevations of cortisol secretion usually do not respond to metyrapone with further increases in total 17-OHCS secretion although there is a qualitative change in adrenal secretion so that the major 17-OHCS is substance S rather than cortisol.

5. Hypopituitarism occurring as a consequence of destruction of the pituitary body is associated with subnormal secretion of ACTH by the pituitary, subnormal secretion of cortisol by the adrenal, and unresponsiveness of the pituitary-adrenal system to stress or metyrapone [28,30]. The functional activity of the system is depressed to such a degree that studies of diurnal rhythmicity and negative feedback suppressibility have little meaning. Adrenal responsiveness to standard test doses of ACTH decreases but can be restored and maintained by prolonged treatment with exogenous ACTH. As soon as exogenous ACTH is withdrawn, however, adrenal atrophy and unresponsiveness recur.

6. Slowly reversible suppression of pituitary-adrenal responsiveness is observed in patients who have received prolonged courses of treatment with supraphysiologic doses of cortisol or those who have had cortisol-secreting adrenal neoplasms. Until the primary excess of cortisol is corrected, ACTH secretion by the pituitary is subnormal, as is cortisol secretion by the nontumorous portions of the adrenal. The course of pituitary-adrenal recovery following the correction of the primary cortisol excess can be described as passing through 3 phases, each of several weeks to several months duration [15].

During the initial phase of recovery, the pituitary secretion of ACTH is subnormal, as is adrenal secretion of cortisol. The pituitary response to metyrapone is negligible, and the adrenal response to a standard test dose of exogenous ACTH is grossly impaired.

During the second phase of recovery, the secretion of ACTH increases to normal and even becomes supernormal, while adrenal secretion of cortisol, although appreciable, remains subnormal. There is a diurnal rhythm in ACTH and cortisol secretion, so that plasma ACTH is distinctly elevated only during the morning and falls to low levels in the evening. Adrenal responsiveness to test doses of ACTH and pituitary-adrenal responses to metyrapone are subnormal.

During the third phase of recovery, adrenal responsiveness to ACTH increases to normal, and plasma ACTH levels fall back to normal. Normal responses to test doses of ACTH and metyrapone are observed. The entire process of pituitary-adrenal recovery usually takes several months if the prior period of continuous profound

GRANT W. LIDDLE

pituitary-adrenal suppression had exceeded a year.

CONCLUDING COMMENTS

It seems to me that we may be approaching the time when there should be a re-appraisal of the usefulness of the concept that the pituitary-adrenal system behaves according to the specifications of a negative feedback regulator. There is no doubt that this has been a very valuable concept in the past in enabling us to describe, explain, and predict the behavior of the system under many different circumstances. It has been one of the powerful abstract concepts in this area of biology and one which I myself have often utilized in designing studies.

However, it has become increasingly apparent in recent years that other factors also influence pituitary-adrenal function in important ways. Major modifications in a negative feedback model must be made if one is to take into account the diurnal rhythmicity and the responsiveness to stress that are exhibited by the normal pituitary-adrenal system. Furthermore, in patients with Cushing's disease and in patients who are recovering from cortisol-induced pituitary-adrenal suppression, the description of the system in terms of a negative-feedback mechanism seems only a rough approximation of the truth.

In the future, I hope we might learn how physicomathematical models can provide better insight into the complex nature of ACTH regulation. Can such models do more than describe data retrospectively? Can they really lead to new insights? It will be interesting to learn whether professional modelers can effectively analyze, criticize, and guide the work of biochemists and neurophysiologists in their efforts to understand the regulation of pituitary-adrenal function.

REFERENCES

1. Bartter, F.C., Albright, F., Forbes, A.P., Leaf, A., Dempsey, E., and Carroll,E. The effects of adrenocorticotropin hormone and cortisone in adrenogenital syndrome associated with congenital adrenal hyperplasia: an attempt to explain and correct its disordered hormonal pattern. *J. Clin. Invest.* 30:237, 1951.

2. Bethune, J.E., Nelson, D.H., and Thorn, G.W. Plasma adrenocorticotrophic hormone in Addison's disease and its modification by administration of adrenal steroids. *J. Clin. Invest.* 36:1701, 1957.

3. Bongiovanni, A.M., and Eberlein, W.R. Defects in steroidal metabolism of subjects with adrenogenital syndrome. *Metabolism* 10:917, 1961.

4. Dexter, R.N., Fishman, L.M., Ney, R.L., and Liddle, G.W. An effect of adreno-corticotropic hormone (ACTH) on adrenal cholesterol accumulation. *Endocrinology* 81:1185, 1967.

5. Doe, R.P., Flink, E.B., and Goodsell, M.G. Relationship of diurnal variation in 17-hydroxycorticosteroid levels in blood and urine to eosinophils and electrolyte excretion. *J. Clin. Endocr. & Metab.* 16:196, 1956.

6. Doe, R.P., Vennes, J.A., and Flink, E.B. Diurnal variation of 17-hydroxycorti-costeroids, sodium, potassium, magnesium, and creatinine and normal subjects and in cases of treated adrenal insufficiency and Cushing's syndrome. *J. Clin. Endocr. & Metab.* 20:253, 1960.

7. Ekman, H., Hakansson, B., McCarthy, J.D., Lehmann, J., and Sjogren, B. Plasma 17-hydroxycorticosteroids in Cushing's syndrome. *J. Clin. Endocr. & Metab.* 21:684, 1961.

8. Estep, H.L., Island, D.P., Ney, R.L., and Liddle, G.W. Pituitary-adrenal dynam-ics during surgical stress. *J. Clin. Endocr. & Metab.* 23:419, 1963.

9. Farese, R.V. Inhibition of steroidogenic effect of ACTH and incorporation of amino acid into rat adrenal protein *in vitro* by chloramphenicol. *Biochem. Biophys. Acta* 87:699, 1964.

10. Ferguson, J.J., Jr. Protein synthesis and adrenocorticotrophin responsiveness. *J. Biol. Chem.* 238:2754, 1963.

11. Forsham, P.H., DiRiamondo, V., Island, D., Rinfret, A.P., and Orr, R.H. Dynamics of adrenal function in man. *Ciba Foundation Colloquia on Endocrinology* 8:279, 1955.

12. Franks, R.C. Diurnal variation of plasma 17-hydroxycorticosteroids in children. *J. Clin. Endocr. & Metab.* 27:75, 1967.

13. Ganong, W.F. The central nervous system and the synthesis and release of adreno-corticotrophic hormone. In *Advances in Neuroendocrinology* (ed. A.V. Nalbandov) University of Illinois Press, Urbana, p. 92, 1963.

14. Garren, L.D., Ney, R.L., and Davis, W.W. Studies on the role or protein syn-thesis in the regulation of corticosterone production by adrenocorticotrophic hormones *in vivo*. *Nat'l. Academy of Sciences Proceedings* 53:1443, 1965.

15. Graber, A.L., Ney, R.L., Nicholson, W.E., Island, D.P., and Liddle, G.W. Natural history of pituitary-adrenal recovery following long-term suppression with cor-ticosteroids. *J. Clin. Endocr. & Metab.* 25:11, 1965.

16. Graber, A.L., Givens, J.R., Nicholson, W.E., Island, D.P., and Liddle, G.W. Per-sistence of diurnal rhythmicity in plasma ACTH concentrations in cortisol-de-ficient patients. *J. Clin. Endocr. & Metab.* 25:804, 1965.

17. Grahame-Smith, D.G., Butcher,R.W., Ney, R.L., and Sutherland, E.W. Adenosine 3', 5'-monophosphate as an intracellular mediator of the action of ACTH on the adrenal cortex. *J. Biol. Chem.* 242:5535, 1967.

18. Haynes, R.C., Jr., and Berthet, L. Studies on mechanism of action of adreno-corticotropic hormone. *J. Biol. Chem.* 225:115, 1957.

GRANT W. LIDDLE

19. Haynes, R.C., Jr. The activation of adrenal phosphorylase by the adrenocorticotropic hormone. *J. Biol. Chem.* 233:1220, 1958

20. Hechter, O., Solomon, M.M., Zaffaroni, A., and Pincus, G. Transformation of cholesterol and acetate to adrenal cortical hormones. *Arch. Biochem.* 46:201, 1953.

21. Hilf, R. The mechanism of action of ACTH. *New Eng. J. Med.* 273:798, 1965.

22. Karaboyas, G.C., and Koritz, S.B. Identity of the site of action of 3', 5'-adenosine monophosphate and adrenocorticotropic hormone in corticosteroidogenesis in rat adrenal and beef adrenal cortex slices. *Biochemistry* 4:462, 1965.

23. Kepler, E.J., Sprague, R.G., Mason, H.L., and Power, M.H. Pathologic physiology of adrenal cortical tumors and Cushing's syndrome. *Rec. Prog. Hormone Res.* 2:345, 1948.

24. Koritz, S.B. Some observations on the stimulation *in vitro* of corticoid production by adenosine 3', 5'-monophosphate in rat adrenals. *Biochim. Biophys. Acta* 60:179, 1962.

25. Krieger, D.T., and Krieger, H.P. Circadian variation of the plasma 17-hydroxycorticosteroids in central nervous system disease. *J. Clin. Endocr. & Metab.* 26:929, 1966.

26. Liddle, G.W., Island, D.P., Rinfret, A.P., and Forsham, P.H. Factors enhancing the response of the human adrenal to corticotropin: is there an adrenal growth factor? *J. Clin. Endocr. & Metab.* 14:839, 1954.

27. Liddle, G.W., Island, D., Lance, E.M., Harris, A.P. Alterations of adrenal steroid patterns in man resulting from treatment with a chemical inhibitor of 11β-hydroxylation. *J. Clin. Endocr. & Metab.* 18:906, 1958.

28. Liddle, G.W., Estep, H.L., Kendall, J.W., Williams, W.C., and Townes, A.W. Clinical application of a new test of pituitary reserve. *J. Clin. Endocr. & Metab.* 19:875, 1959.

29. Liddle, G.W. Tests of adrenocortical reserve, pituitary reserve, and pituitary-adrenal suppressibility. In *Clinical Endocrinology* 1 (ed. E.B. Astwood) Grune and Stratton, Inc., New York, p. 672, 1960.

30. Liddle, G.W., Island, D.P., and Meador, C.,. Normal and Abnormal regulation of corticotropin secretion in man. *Rec. Prog. Hormone Res.* 18:125, 1962.

31. Liddle, G.W., Island, D.P., Ney, R.L., Nicholson, W.E., and Shimizu, N. Non-pituitary neoplasms and Cushing's syndrome. *Archives of Int. Med.* 111:471, 1963.

32. Liddle, G.W., Givens, J.R., Nicholson, W.E., and Island, D.P. The ectopic ACTH syndrome. *Cancer Res.* 25:1057, 1965.

33. Liddle, G.W. An analysis of circadian rhythms in human adrenocortical secretory activity. *Arch. Int. Med.* 117:739, 1966.

34. Lindsay, A.E., Migeon, C.J., Nugent, C.A., and Brown, H. The diagnostic value of plasma and urinary 17-hydroxycorticosteroid determinations in Cushing's syndrome. *Amer. J. Med.* 20:15, 1956.

35. Mason, J.W. Psychological influences on the pituitary-adrenal cortical system. *Rec. Prog. Hormone Res.* 15:345, 1959.

36. McKerns, K.W. Mechanism of action of adrenocorticotropic hormone through activation of glucose-6-phosphate dehydrogenase. *Biochim. Biophys. Acta* 90:357, 1964.

37. Meador, C.K., Liddle, G.W., Island, D.P., Nicholson, W.E., Lucas, C.P., Nuckton, J.G., and Luetscher, J.A. Cause of Cushing's syndrome in patients with tumors arising from "nonendocrine" tissue. *J. Clin. Endocr. & Metab.* 22:693, 1962.

38. Ney, R.L., Shimizu, N., Nicholson, W.E., Island, D.P., and Liddle, G.W. correlation of plasma ACTH concentration with adrenocortical response in normal human subjects, surgical patients, and patients with Cushing's disease. *J. Clin. Invest.* 42:1669, 1963.

39. Ney, R.L., Dexter, R.N., Davis, W.W., and Garren, L.D. A study of the mechanisms by which adrenocorticotropic hormone maintains adrenal steroidogenic responsiveness. *J. Clin. Invest.* 46:1916, 1967.

40. Nichols, C.T., and Tyler, F.H. Diurnal variation in adrenal cortical function. *Ann. Rev. Med.* 18:313, 1967.

41. Nugent, C.A., Eik-Nes, K., Samuels, L.T., and Tyler, F.H. Changes in plasma levels of 17-hydroxycorticosteroids during the intravenous administration of adrenocorticotropin (ACTH). IV. Response to prolonged infusions of small amounts of ACTH. *J. Clin. Endocr. & Metab.* 19:334, 1959.

42. Orth, D.N., Island, D.P., and Liddle, G.W. Experimental alteration of the circadian rhythm in plasma cortisol (17-OHCS) concentration in man. *J. Clin. Endocr. & Metab.* 27:549, 1967.

43. Paris, J. Pituitary-adrenal suppression after protracted administration of adrenal cortical hormones. *Proc. Mayo Clinic* 36:305, 1961.

44. Perkoff, G.T., Eik-Nes, K., Nugent, C.A., Fred, H.L., Nimer, R.A., Rush, L., Samuels, L.T., and Tyler, F.H. Studies of the diurnal variation of plasma 17-hydroxycorticosteroids in man. *J. Clin. Endocr. & Metab.* 19:432, 1959.

45. Pincus, G. Diurnal rhythm in excretion of urinary ketosteroids by young men. *J. Clin. Endocr. & Metab.* 3:195, 1943.

46. Saba, N., Hechter, O., and Stone, D. The conversion of cholesterol to pregnenolone in bovine adrenal homogenates. *J. Amer. Chem. Soc.* 76:3862, 1954.

47. Sayers, G., and Royce, P.C. Regulation of the secretory activity of the adrenal cortex. In *Clinical Endocrinology* 1 (ed. E.B. Astwood) Grune and Stratton, Inc., New York, p. 323, 1960.

48. Schwartz, T.B. Adrenal hyperresponsiveness resulting from prolonged corticotropin therapy. *J. Clin. Endocr. & Metab.* 19:269, 1959.

49. Sydnor, K.L., Kelley, V.C., Raile, R.B., Ely, R.S., and Sayers, G. Blood adrenocorticotropin in children with congenital adrenal hyperplasia. *Proc. Soc. Exper. Biol. & Med.* 82:695, 1953.

50. Takebe, K., Setaishi, C., Hirama, M., Yamamoto, M., and Horiuciti, Y. Effects of a bacterial pyrogen on the pituitary-adrenal axis at various times in the 24 hours. *J. Clin. Endocr. & Metab.* 26:437, 1966.

51. Taylor, A.B., Albert, A., and Sprague, R.G. Adrenotrophic activity of human blood. *Endocrinology* 45:335, 1949.

52. Urquhart, J., and Li, C.C. The dynamics of adrenocortical secretion. *Amer. J. Physiol.* (in press).

53. Wilkins, L., Bongiovanni, A.M., Clayton, G.W., Grumbach, M.M., and Van Wyk, J. Virilizing adrenal hyperplasia: its treatment with cortisone and the nature of the steroid abnormalities. *Ciba Found. Coll. on Endocrinology: The Human Adrenal Cortex* 8:460, 1955.

GRANT W. LIDDLE

54. Williams, W.C., Island, D.P., Oldfield, R.A.A., and Liddle, G.W. Blood corti-
     cotropin (ACTH) levels in Cushing's disease. *J. Clin. Endocr. & Metab.* 21:426,
     1961.

55. Zukoski, C.F. Mechanism of action of insulin hypoglycemia on adrenal cortical
     secretion. *Endocrinology* 78:1264, 1966.

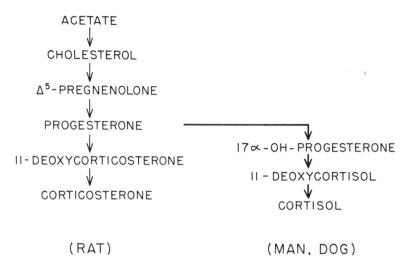

FIG. 1.   Some of the major steps in the corticosteroid biosynthetic pathway.

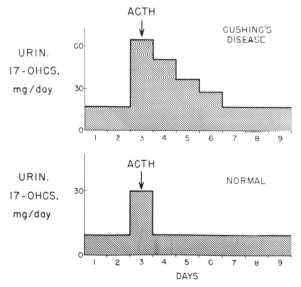

FIG. 2.   Typical responses to an 8-hour intravenous infusion of 50 units of ACTH in a normal subject (lower) and in a patient with Cushing's disease (upper).

F.E. YATES and R.D. BRENNAN
Department of Physiology, Stanford University, Stanford, California; IBM Scientific Center, Palo Alto, California

2. STUDY OF THE MAMMALIAN ADRENAL GLUCOCORTICOID SYSTEM BY COMPUTER SIMULATION

INTRODUCTION

Attempts to simulate complicated biological systems by means of computer models immediately pose philosophical as well as practical problems. The philosophical problems concern the nature of models and the act of modeling. Although presumably all biologists use some form of symbolic abstraction (words, diagrams, gestures) when they consider the systems of interest to them, many nevertheless are skeptical about the value of computer simulation in biology. Their skepticism surprisingly may exceed that with which they regard verbal constructs or diagrams. In our opinion, advantages and strengths of computer simulation as a means to express understanding of complex biological systems are the following:

1. Computer simulations (models) of biological systems require that the static and dynamic characteristics of all the pertinent components and processes of the systems be identified and quantitatively specified;

2. Computer models are truly functional – they can change state with the flow of time, and therefore they expose the incompleteness of knowledge. They also reveal contradicitons that may characterize the notions of even a very competent scientist who tries to explain a system so complex that his unaided intuition fails to perceive all the consequences of his many assertions and beliefs about it.

---

*The experimental work and modeling done by us was supported by USPHS Grant AM 04612 and Life Insurance Medical Research Fund Grant G-66-23-02 to Dr. F.E. Yates.

F.E. YATES AND R.D. BRENNAN

The attempt to accomplish a computer simulation of a biological system can be very humbling. It is a common discovery in such attempts that the data available are of little use because the experiments from which they came were not designed or executed to answer quantitative questions about system dynamics. This discovery can be sharply unpleasant. Nevertheless, we believe that the strongest proof of "understanding" of a complex biological system consists of the successful simulation of the system by means of a computer model. Therefore we regard successful simulation as a necessary objective of mature physiological systems work.

Successful Simulation

Computer simulations in biology consist of mathematical or logical programs describing a biological system, that are interpretable by the chosen computer so that experimental or artificial data are accepted as parameters, initial conditions and inputs, and the values of all the relevant state or algebraic variables of the system are given as functions of time for the outputs. The output solutions obtained by the computer with either type of data are then compared with the solutions obtained from analogous experiments on the chosen biological system.

Judgments about the success of a simulation (model) are based upon two considerations:

1. The fit of the computer outputs to those given by the biological system itself for analogous experiments must be adequate. No general criterion of adequacy of fit in such cases can be hoped for, and the modeler is left to decide for himself whether or not the fit has been adequate. The inescapable subjectiveness of such judgments gives a proper cause to distrust modelers—but not to distrust the act of modeling itself.

2. The model must be constrained as far as existing information allows by having its structure based upon the identifiable unit processes of the real biological system. This point deserves further explanation because it concerns the lack of uniqueness of models. Although biological systems necessarily perform in some unique, particular way (their design is already given) it is always possible to simulate any selected, observed performance in more than one way. Nevertheless, as more and more different observations are simulated by a single model, the model matures by becoming progressively more constrained and more powerful as predictor of performance of the biological system in experiments that are feasible but

not yet performed. Thus, with increasing maturation a model evolves from a formal model (i.e., one that simulates observed functions by any means whatever capable of producing adequate fit to describe <u>what</u> the system does) - toward the ultimate, isomorphic and unique model (unattainable) that describes exactly and particularly <u>how</u> the system does it. An isomorphic model would have perfect predictive power.

In some cases a biologist may desire only to make a formal model, adequate for simulation of a restricted set of performance characteristics. He could use such a limited model empirically for the purposes of diagnosis and therapy in clinical medicine, as in the case of predicting insulin requirements from plasma glucose levels in diabetics by means of a formal model of glucose metabolism. For this use the model could be judged successful if it satisfied only the first, but not the second consideration given above. Such an application of a formal model represents a worthwhile engineering achievement but, for the purposes of understanding how systems work, models must be judged successful in proportion to the degree that they have matured from the formal toward the isomorphic kind.

In our opinion, it is confusion between formal and isomorphic models, and failure to recognize the great differences in the criteria appropriate for judgment of success of a model for engineering purposes as opposed to scientific purposes, that together are responsible for many of the apparent disagreements about philosophies of modeling in biology.

Elsewhere we have discussed in greater detail the philosophy and strategy of modeling in biology, as well as the practical difficulties involved [38]. In this present paper we shall present a model of the adrenocortical glucocorticoid neuroendocrine system in sufficient detail so that it can be put into operation by anyone with access to either a digital or an analog computer of appropriate capacity. We hope that by so doing we will permit this model to be easily used, and subsequently judged, modified and improved. It seems to us to be important that models be readily communicated among interested scientists. This must be so if models are to serve to advance the field of which they are a part, rather than merely to give private esthetic satisfaction to their originators.

Documentation of the Model

The model to be presented is based upon an extensive literature in the field of adrenocortical physiology that began in the 1930's. Six **discussions that include** much of the work which we have now incorporated into the present model may be found in review articles [5,6,15,25,35,37]. Yamamoto and Raub [33] have pointed out, however, that it is difficult to evaluate a model if review articles or books or other secondary sources are used as documentation. They believe that a model should be judged according to the adequacy with which it can be shown to simulate the primary data claimed to have been used in its construction, and in addition, according to the adequacy with which it simulates other existing, relevant primary data not immediately used in the construction of the model. Finally, it should be judged according to its ability to predict new data obtainable from feasible experiments performed after development of the model.

We believe the above views have merit, but we shall compromise to avoid re-reviewing the field here, and use existing reviews for indirect documentation with older relevant work, whereas we shall cite or present some very recent primary data as examples of more direct documentation of the model.

History of the Current Model

The current model has evolved slowly, and various stages of its development have been previously presented. In chronological order the previous forms have evolved from hydraulic analog [28], verbal construct [34], differential equations for the steady-state [35], analog computer model [37], to a digital computer model based upon state equations embodying transient responses as well as steady-state performance, using a digital analog simulation language [38]. The present model is of the same type as that given recently in reference 38, but it is more comprehensive and will be described here in more detail than has been used for the earlier versions.

Computer Program Used for the Present Model

The 1130 Continuous System Modeling Program (1130 CSMP) for the IBM 1130 computer was used for the model. We have given a brief description of this program elsewhere [38], and the IBM program reference manual may be consulted for fuller description [9]. The symbolic notation for the operations available in this program that were used in the model is shown in Figure 1. Although the symbols resemble those used for analog computer programs, they differ in that the electronic constraints of sign-reversal with analog computer summer or intergrator elements, as well as the voltage overload protection provided through division by the maximum voltage of the analog computer when analog multipliers are used, are not required in this program. Thus the symbols in Figure 1 refer only to the indicated operations, and do not imply that there is any other concealed operation such as sign reversal. In 1130 CSMP,

MAMMALIAN ADRENAL GLUCOCORTICOID SYSTEM

variables are given their proper signs by designating the sign along with the numbers used to set the constant multipliers, constant source, constant initial conditions or other parameters. To translate the computer diagrams presented in this paper to an analog computer program it is necessary to add a sign reversal amplifier (multiplication by -1) at the output of the summers and intergrators, and to scale the multipliers to prevent overloading in the usual fashion for analog computers [10].

The functions indicated in Figure 1 are described in sufficient detail to permit construction from analog computer elements, if desired. For the users of other digital analog simulation languages, the translation from 1130 CSMP will be possible directly from the computer diagrams to be shown, and from the description of special and other functions indicated in Figure 1.

In addition to the computer simulation diagrams shown in the body of this paper, we have presented a complete configuration listing giving the connectivity of the model in a more convenient form for programming, as well as a complete listing of the numerical values with signs for all the initial conditions, sources, and parameters in the model. Finally, we have also presented the algebraic and state equations that specify the model.

THE ADRENAL GLUCOCORTICOID SYSTEM MODEL

The Configuration of the Adrenal Glucocorticoid System

The general organization of the mammalian adrenal glucocorticoid system is presented in Figure 2. The various gross features of the organization of this system are as follows:

1.   Multiple anatomically **distinct** pathways in the brain can stimulate the adrenocortical system. The pathways are represented as positive inputs to the system in Figure 2.

2.   Some neural pathways, possibly involving the hippocampus, may inhibit the adrenocortical system. Such a pathway is shown as a negative input in Figure 2.

3.   The brain (hypothalamic median eminence) stimulates the synthesis and secretion of corticotropin (ACTH) at the adenohypophysis (pituitary) by means of a neurohormone, corticotropin-releasing factor (CRF), that is conveyed to the pituitary by the blood flow through the hypothalamic-pituitary portal vessels.

4. ACTH enters the general systemic circulation and is distributed throughout the extracellular fluid of the body, and is bound by some tissues, (e.g., kidney). ACTH is rapidly metabolized, and may be adsorbed by components in the blood. The distribution, binding and metabolism processes for ACTH are specified by the ACTH D.B.M. element in Figure 2.

5. ACTH stimulates synthesis and secretion of androgenic, estrogenic, mineralocorticoid (aldosterone) (only transiently) and glucocorticoid (corticosterone, cortisol) hormones and some of their precursors from the adrenal cortex. The system to be modeled is the glucocorticoid system, so only two outputs (cortisol and corticosterone) are indicated as secretion rates in Figure 2. ACTH also causes an enlargement of the adrenal cortex, over a long time scale, and also may increase the sensitivity of the secretion rate response to ACTH. These parametric effects are shown by the input at the bottom of the adrenal cortex element in Figure 2. ACTH acts on the brain over a long period to inhibit some responses of the adrenocortical system (dashed loop in Figure 2). The sensitivity of the adrenocortical secretory response to ACTH is dependent upon adrenal blood flow, as indicated by the parametric blood flow input in Figure 2.

6. Glucocorticoids are distributed throughout the extracellular fluid, and are bound to two plasma proteins, albumin and a globulin (called transcortin in humans). The hormones are metabolized primarily by the liver, but also by other tissues and organs. The rate of metabolism is dependent upon hepatic blood flow, and upon thyroid and possibly also gonadal steroid hormone levels. The levels of the binding globulin can be increased by thyroid or estrogenic hormones.

7. Glucocorticoid target tissues are affected by unbound glucocorticoids (c_{GLUC}).

8. The unbound glucocorticoids act on at least four separate sites in the brain, and possibly also upon the adenohypophysis (pituitary) to inhibit the system. This inhibitory action is represented as a multistage negative feedback loop in Figure 2.

Extensive documentation of these general properties of the glucocorticoid system may be found in several review articles [5,6,15,25,35,37].

MAMMALIAN ADRENAL GLUCOCORTICOID SYSTEM

Reduced Configuration of the System as Modeled

The present model is intended to characterize the acute, immediate responses of the adrenocortical glucocorticoid system to sudden perturbation. The relevant time domain for the model is approximately four hours or less, and all properties of the system that appear or change over a longer time scale are omitted from the model. The multiple inputs and multistage feedback sites in the central nervous system are reduced to two each, and the pituitary feedback stage is omitted because it is not yet clear whether or not it operates within the physiological range of glucocorticoid hormone levels. The multiple outputs of the adrenal cortex have been reduced to a single output, representing the dominant glucocorticoid hormone (cortisol for most species). The reduced configuration that served as a basis for the model is shown in Figure 3.

Species Modeled

The gross configuration of the adrenal glucocorticoid system so far appears to be the same in all mammalian species studied. We have chosen to scale the model for a 15 kg, lean dog, with a blood volume of 1.2 liters, and a plasma volume of 0.69 liters (0.042 L/kg; whole body hematocrit = 44%). Normal resting total adrenal blood flow was taken as 8 ml/min. Qualitative information supporting the configuration of the model has come from studies on man, rat, and dog.

The Problem of Real Individuals and Distorted Averages

From individual dogs and humans it is often feasible to obtain sequential samples during a response of the adrenocortical system to some stimulus. Data from each individual yield a curve showing the variable of interest as a function of time. If a population of such individual curves is obtained during an experimental study, and these curves differ in amplitudes and time relationships, the problem arises of how best to represent the experimental data in a model. The simple technique of averaging the data can distort the responses severely. For example, it is obvious that a population of pure sine waves of common amplitude but various frequencies would yield a periodic function that is not a sine wave if at each point in time the amplitudes are averaged to generate the curve supposed to be representative of the population of data. In this case the "average" curve is not at all representative of the true wave form.

In experiments on rats and other very small animals, when the time course of a

F.E.YATES AND R.D. BRENNAN

response is being studied, individual animals usually contribute only a single datum at one point in time, rather than an individual curve. The desired functional relationship is then obtained by joining the means of data from populations of animals studied at different times. The resulting curve is representative of some fictional "average" animal. This average is clearly different from the distorted average obtained for populations of curves, as described above, but is it any more representative? These common features of dynamic studies in biology present difficulties for the system modeler.

Since we do not usually introduce noise **deliberately** into deterministic models (though it might be wise to do so), continuous **system** models such as the one to be described below are truly deterministic: they give exactly the same response each time they are forced in the same way. We must then ask what the response represents—that of some plausible individual from the population of animals studied, or that of a mythical "average" animal, whose averaged responses may not represent even the shapes of the true responses in the experimental population?

For the present work we decided upon the following arbitrary technique for dealing with the problem of finding representative data to use in simulation of system dynamics. We first separated the shapes of curves from their amplitudes by normalization. For example, if the curves went through some maximu, or reached some final steady-state constant value, or had some non-zero initial condition, we attempted to express the curves with each datum as a fraction of the chosen reference value, which was set to 1.0. Variable delays, if any, were then subtracted by shifting the time scale for each curve so the onsets of the dynamic responses appeared to be simultaneous. The data were then averaged at each point in time so an average normalized curve resulted. This curve was taken to have a shape representative of the population of shapes for the purposes of developing the model.

To obtain a representative amplitude scale, some feature of the curves (e.g., a maximum, a plateau, etc.) were averaged, regardless of slight differences in times of occurrence, and this averaged amplitude was assigned to the same feature of the average normalized curve obtained as described above. The ordinate scale was thus converted to representative absolute values. This final curve was adopted for the purposes of modeling, and was considered to be usefully representative of the data, after an averaged delay was introduced if variable delays had been present in the raw data.

It would be possible to use parameter optimization techniques according to some criterion such as can be found in nonlinear least squares curve fitting programs [12], to obtain the representative curve used for modeling, but this and other statistical techniques still force a decision about what is meant by "representative" when system

MAMMALIAN ADRENAL GLUCOCORTICOID SYSTEM

dynamics for a highly variable population of individuals are under consideration.
Yamamoto and Raub [33], pointed out that no agreed upon standard technique for decid-
ing whether a model fits data has been achieved. We have described our crude and
arbitrary method to give emphasis to the problem. In several instances we will present experimental data, with documentation of source, that have been fitted by the
computer model. Because of application of the normalization and ordinate scaling
techniques described above, the data are not shown exactly as they were published.
In some cases the effects of our normalization and scaling were very slight, as when
the raw data had little variation; in other cases the effect was large, and the data
cannot easily be identified exactly in the original source without taking account of
our method of scaling. For that reason we have cited the individual Figures and
Tables of the references used to supply the primary data.

Decomposition of the System into Subsystems for Modeling

We shall describe in sequence the following subsystems of the complete adrenal
glucocorticoid system in detail:

I.   Cortisol distribution, binding and metabolism processes
II. Cortisol secretory response of the adrenal to ACTH input
III. Central elements
    a.   ACTH distribution and metabolism processes
    b.   ACTH secretory response of the pituitary to CRF input
    c.   Relation between neural inputs and CRF release
    d.   Feedback comparator action
    e.   Feedback path characteristics

Each subsystem model will be developed and presented in six steps:

1. Diagram of the subsystem configuration
2. State or algebraic equations defining the model
3. Diagram of computer representation of the model equations
4. Table of configuration listings for the computer diagram
5. Tuning of parameters from data; scaling
6. Table listing initial conditions (IC) and parameters of
    the scaled subsystem models.

By this means a very complete specification of the model can be achieved so that it can be used by the reader if he desires.

Variables and Parameters of the Model

The variables of the model are listed in Table I, with their symbols and units of measurements. These variables are time-variant quantities defined either by differential equations (in which case they are state variables and appear at the outputs of integrators in the model) or by algebraic, integrated equations, (in which case they appear at the outputs of the other types of elements in the model).

The parameters of the model are listed in Table II, with their symbols, units, and their numerical values estimated for normal scaling of the model for a 15 kg dog. The justification of these values will appear in the discussion of each subsystem below. Table III lists 8 parameters that appear in the equations, but that are not shown explicitly in the computer diagrams either because they have unity value, or because they have been subsumed into other composite parameters.

The parameters of the model are quantities that may change slowly in time during the life of a dog, but which are time-invariant within the time domain of relevance of the model (4 hours or less).

Experimental Inputs and Parametric Forcing Functions

The model may be forced by 9 inputs, singly or in combination. These are shown in Table IV. They appear in the computer diagrams as constants or constant sources that may have zero or positive values, except for the inhibitory morphine input, which may have zero or negative values. Thus, as the model is shown, the inputs are restricted to step function forcing. However, it is obvious that these inputs could be separately driven by any other functions deemed appropriate. We have shown the arrangements for step forcing because they are the simplest, and the most commonly used in the initial exploration of the performance of a model. The justification for showing the basal level circadian rhythm input as a constant is that during most four-hour time domains, circadian trends are not conspicuous. Obviously the very rapid circadian drive of the system that may occur between 4 to 8 a.m. in normal humans, or between 4 to 8 p.m. in the nocturnal rat would require nonconstant representation.

Two parametric forcing functions in the model are also shown in Table IV.

MAMMALIAN ADRENAL GLUCOCORTICOID SYSTEM

Initial Conditions and Baseline Performance of the Model: Model Time Domain

Unilateral adrenocortical secretion rates in unanesthetized dogs, measured 3 to
5 days after right adrenalectomy and preparation for intermittent collection of left
adrenal venous outflow by the method of Hume and Nelson, [8] are usually very low and
close to the residual value observed after hypophysectomy (Table V). It appears that
the baseline, initial conditions of the dog adrenocortical system are nearly zero.
A baseline circadian rhythm has been difficult to define in the dog [7,13]. Curve C
of Figure 4 shows a circadian study of dog No. 2 from Table V. Only three cortisol
secretion rate values of the 18 obtained over a 25 hour period lie above 0.4 µg/min.
Although the two bursts of ACTH release implied by the curve, at 10 a.m. and 6 a.m.
on successive mornings, might represent a basal periodicity in the unstimulated system, it is more likely that the dog was stimulated in an unknown manner at these two
times. Other animals have shown occasional aperiodic spikes in cortisol secretion
rate, usually accompanied by an increase in heart rate, even though no experimental
perturbation of the system was attempted. We interpret these data as indicating that
this endocrine system in the dog has nearly zero initial conditions at all times of
the day if the system is undisturbed.

In the studies to be described that were performed with the model, the initial
conditions were set slightly higher than zero. Since the model was designed to simulate acute responses of the adrenocortical system, we did not require or expect that
it would match the performance of the system in the dog over a longer time period.
Of course, this model can serve as the basis for an extended version that does simulate both acute and longer-term performance of the real system, and such an extension is under development. However, the present version of the model is intended to
simulate only responses that are short-term (up to four hours) in duration after a
stimulus. In fact, if our model is used for a longer simulation period, its performance may depart from that of the real system (compare curves B and C, Figure 4).

Because work on the rat had indicated that the feedback path for corticosteroids
has a two hour delay in it [3], such a delay was included in the present model for
the dog. We have introduced the assumption that the adrenocortical system has the
same configuration in all mammalian species, and that the various species differ
only in the values of the system parameters. This assumption requires additional
testing by means of comparative studies, but from the available evidence, it seems
to be a reasonable assumption. The two-hour delay has not been looked for in the
dog. Nevertheless, we have included it so that our model will have general usefulness for simulation of adrenocortical system data from rat, man or dog with appropriate scaling for each species. The delay can easily be suppressed in the general

model. When it is present in the model scaled for the dogs, and the initial conditions are greater than zero, a steady-state baseline oscillation, with a period of approximately six hours, and a higher **frequency** underdamped oscillation, with a period of approximately nine minutes are both present (Figure 4). If the two-hour feedback delay is removed, the slower oscillation disappears.

The model must run for the computer equivalent of 300 minutes of experimental time (which is approximately 15 minutes, since the computer model runs about 20 times faster than does the real system it simulates), before it enters the true steady-state initial conditions oscillation. This initial period is required because at the outset the digit delay element stores only an arbitrary constant: it cannot store a periodic function as initial condition. One cycle has to occur before the delay element is properly generating a correct periodic signal equal to the value of its varying input two hours earlier. These features of the model are illustrated in curves A and B, Figure 4.

Many of the experiments on the model to be presented lasted only for the equivalent of 120 minutes of real experimental time, or less, so the delay element was not functioning during them as a variable signal element, but rather as a constant.

It is not yet known whether the dog adrenocortical system has the periodicity shown in Figure 4 when it is driven steadily by a small step input analogous to that used for the initial conditions of the model. Consequently, at the present time we emphasize the usefulness of the complete model only for simulation of adrenocortical responses in the period of two hours after acute perturbation. Whether the model is appropriate for simulation of experimental data obtained over longer periods remains to be seen. However, the model component for the cortisol distribution, binding and metabolism subsystem has been validated in isolation for a four-hour period, as will be shown.

Integration Interval

The integration interval used in all cases was 0.25 minutes (simulation time). If an interval greater than 0.4 minutes is used, the accuracy of the simulation degenerates during rapid transient responses. At the 0.25 minute integration interval, the model runs 20 times faster than real experimental time. This rather small value for the speed-up of experimental time stems from the large number of integrations in the complete model that have to be performed serially. The slight disadvantage of slowness of the model on the IBM 1130 computer is compensated by the availability of frequent and precise printout of values of all the selected variables at chosen times during a run, so that the graphical outputs are very well documented by digital data.

MAMMALIAN ADRENAL GLUCOCORTICOID SYSTEM

SUBSYSTEM I: CORTISOL DISTRIBUTION, BINDING AND METABOLISM PROCESSES

Extensive documentation of the main features of the corticosteroid distribution, binding and metabolism processes may be found in several review sources [14,21,26,35]. The corticosteroids are secreted into the blood in unbound form, and are then absorbed by albumin and a specific globulin (transcortin) and by erythrocytes. An equilibrium distribution is believed to be present in arterial blood. Both unbound and protein-bound corticosteroids pass through capillary walls (at very different rates) by diffusion and filtration, and a new equilibrium distribution among the three forms (unbound, albumin-bound, and globulin-bound) is present in interstitial fluids. Corticosteroids penetrate cells, and are possibly adsorbed within cells. Some enterohepatic circulation of unmetabolized corticosteroids may be present. The corticosteroids are enzymatically converted to inactive or less active compounds mainly by the liver, but also by some other tissues.

A complete representation of the processes of distribution, binding, and metabolism would require the use of partial differential equations, in which corticosteroid concentrations were continuous functions of both space and time. Since the geometry of the capillary bed, and various interstitial fluids and intracellular domains are not precisely known, the compartmental hypothesis is introduced [23], in which corticosteroid concentrations are regarded as discontinuous functions of space, but continuous functions of time. Thus a distributed system is converted to a lumped system. Such a procedure leads to great simplification of mathematical treatment, and is acceptable as long as no important time relationships (e.g., dispersions) in the real distributed system are distorted or lost in the lumped approximation. In the case of the glucocorticoid system, the compartmental hypothesis leads to excellent simulation, as will be shown.

The possible number of compartments that might be relevant in the lumped system is seven or more [14,36]. Fortunately, however, the subsystem can be effectively represented by the operations indicated in Figure 5, and these can be further lumped in the case of man and dog into the compartmental configuration in Figure 6. This configuration has been used by Nugent et al, as the basis of simulation of cortisol dynamics in humans [17], and we have adapted their model for the dog.

F.E. YATES AND R.D. BRENNAN

Equations

The equations of the subsystem model are:

Conservation of cortisol mass in plasma
1)

$$V_1 \frac{d(C_{c.P})}{dt} = \dot{Q}_c + \dot{Q}_{c.i} - k_{10}(C_{c.P}) - V_1 \frac{d(C_{cT.P})}{dt} - V_1 \frac{d(C_{cA.P})}{dt} - V_2 \frac{d(C_{c.2})}{dt}$$

2)

$$\Sigma\, C_{c.P} = C_{c.P} + C_{cA.P} + C_{cT.P}$$

Conservation of cortisol mass in outer compartment:

3)

$$V_2 \frac{d(C_{c.2})}{dt} = k_{12}\,(C_{c.P}) - k_{21}\,(C_{c.2})$$

Conservation of transcortin in plasma:

4)

$$\Sigma\, C_{T.P} = C_{cT.P} + C_{T.P}$$

Conservation of albumin in plasma:

5)

$$\Sigma\, C_{A.P} = C_{cA.P} + C_{A.P}$$

Reversible binding of cortisol to transcortin (bi-molecular reaction):

6)

$$V_1 \frac{d(C_{cT.P})}{dt} = k_{Ta}(C_{c.P})(C_{T.P}) - k_{Tr}\,(C_{cT.P})$$

Reversible binding of cortisol to albumin (uni-molecular reaction):

MAMMALIAN ADRENAL GLUCOCORTICOID SYSTEM

7)

$$V_1 \frac{d(C_{cA.P})}{dt} = k_{Aa}(C_{c.P}) - k_{Ar}(C_{cA.P})$$

Negative clipping: limiting of reactant concentrations to zero or positive values only:

8)

$$\Sigma \, C_{T.P} - C_{cT.P} \geqslant 0$$

(This equation limits the transcortin variables; when they are so limited, all other variables in the subsystem are implicitly limited also, and no further explicit negative clipping is required.)

Assumptions Behind the Subsystem Equations

The above equations embody the following major assumptions [17]:

a. The adsorption of cortisol by albumin may be represented as a uni-molecular reaction because the concentration of unassociated albumin sites for cortisol is so large that changes in $C_{A.P}$ can be ignored, and $C_{A.P}$ can be included in the constant k_{Aa}.

b. The many extravascular compartments for cortisol may be lumped as one uniform compartment, so that all cortisol in the lumped extravascular compartment may be effectively represented as existing at a single concentration that acts thermodynamically as the activity of cortisol in the outer compartment, regardless of the degree of any binding cortisol in the outer compartment.

c. The disposal of cortisol from the body, which occurs by several different processes, may be represented by a single lumped process, that is first-order with respect to $C_{c.P}$.

Computer Simulation Diagram; Configuration Listing

The configuration of Figure 6 and the eight equations are programmed as shown in Figure 7. The configuration listing specifying the program in Figure 7 is given in Table VI.

Evaluation of Parameters from Data

As a first approximation, the parameters used by Nugent, et al for the human were adjusted for a 15 kg lean dog on a proportional basis. The time base was changed from hours to minutes. Data from the equilibrium binding curve for the dog previously published [21] were fitted by adjusting the total concentration of transcortin parameter of the model, when the model was reduced to simulate such in vitro experiments by setting k_{10} and k_{12} both to zero. An excellent fit of the data could be obtained (Figure 8). From the model and the parameters providing the fit, the dog corticosteroid binding proteins were found to have the following physiochemical characteristics:

Binding Protein	Association Constant (L/M)	Total Concentration of Cortisol Binding Sites (M/L)
"Transcortin"	2.4×10^{7}	2.8×10^{-7}
"Albumin"	3.2×10^{3}	0.5×10^{-3}

Three of these parameters are essentially the same as those for human plasma, but the total concentration of transcortin binding sites in dog plasma is only about 40 per cent of the level in human plasma.

The clearance coefficients defining the metabolic clearance rate of cortisol, and its exchange between inner and outer compartments were obtained by fitting the cortisol disappearance curve data for adrenalectomized dogs published by Thomasson and Steenburg (mean values of Table 3 of Reference [27]). In the experiments by Thomasson and Steenburg, cortisol was determined by a reasonably specific method. However, no data were obtained in the early minutes of pulse injection of cortisol at a dose of 2 mg/kg i.v. Furthermore, the total extra-adrenal pool of cortisol in dogs weighing approximately 10 kg is only 2.0 mg [22], so the dose used by these investigators was large for dogs. As a result, the plasma levels of cortisol were high, and well above the rather low physiological maximum of about 150 µg/L observed in this species.

MAMMALIAN ADRENAL GLUCOCORTICOID SYSTEM

The fit of the data shown in Figure 9 was obtained by adjusting the remaining parameters of the model of Nugent et al, after the parameters of the protein binding reactions had been set by the previous data. After the clearance coefficient for the removal of cortisol (k_{10} in the present model) was increased 20 per cent and the value of V_2 was increased by 33 per cent from the values used in the model for humans, the fit of the data from dogs was good, as shown in the Figure.

The values for all the parameters of the subsystem model, as well as the initial conditions present when the subsystem is connected to the complete model are listed in Table VII.

The subsystem model has other properties also known to be present in the real system. For example, Figure 10 shows that in the model the shape of a cortisol disappearance curve is dependent upon the size of the pulse injection of cortisol. When data from experiments with different doses are plotted in normalized fashion, it can be seen that the largest dose leaves the plasma more rapidly (because it saturates transcortin more effectively) than does the lowest dose.

Eventually, disappearance curves all can be approximately described by a terminal, single exponential decay. This terminal decay can be used to estimate a half-life, although the value obtained is not a simple function of the parameters of the system, and so it has limited usefulness. However, since it is commonly measured, its dependence upon the initial dose of cortisol used, as well as upon transcortin levels have been tested in the model. The results are shown in Table VIII. The terminal half-life for cortisol increases with increasing dose. It is well known that in the real system tracer dose experiments give shorter half-lives than do pharmacological dose experiments [18,19,20,35]. The terminal half-life also increases with increasing transcortin levels [16,26,35] and the model shows this effect also.

The subsystem model is non-linear as demonstrated by the data in both Figures 10 and 11. Figure 11 shows that the Superposition Principle defining linear systems does not hold for cortisol distribution, binding and metabolism processes. If a constant infusion of cortisol is used to elevate plasma cortisol levels, the final level achieved in the steady-state is not doubled when the infusion rate is doubled. The real corticosteroid distribution, binding and metabolism processes have this non-linear property [3,17].

F.E. YATES AND R.D. BRENNAN

SUBSYSTEM II: CORTISOL SECRETORY RESPONSE OF THE ADRENAL TO ACTH INPUT

The dynamic and static properties of isolated, perfused canine adrenal glands, with respect to the cortisol secretory response to ACTH have been studied in great detail by Urquhart and Li [30,31,32]. From their work, and previous work which they review, it appears that the response has the following dominant features:

1. The effective input concentration range for ACTH in whole arterial blood is 0 to 100 mU/L.

2. The onset of adrenal secretory response to a change in ACTH levels is delayed two minutes.

3. A step increase in ACTH in the lower dose range (0-10 mU/L leads to an overshooting adrenal response that reaches a peak in 10 minutes that is 65 percent greater than the steady-state secretion rate achieved about 30 minutes after the input change. The overshoot is not present if the gland is restimulated within five minutes after removal of the input, but it reappears upon restimulation if a longer recovery period is allowed.

4. When ACTH step inputs are reduced in a stepwise fashion, no undershoot occurs (the gland is dynamically assymmetrical) and the decreases in secretion rate follow a monotonic exponential decay with a time constant of three minutes.

5. Up to the point of maximum response, the steady-state secretion rate outputs are a non-linear function of steady ACTH inputs, such that the output is approximately proportional to the logarithm of the input.

6. The adrenal has a low residual secretion of cortisol in the absence of an ACTH input.

7. The steady-state adrenal response to ACTH is increased at increased blood flows, in the low ACTH input range.

8. The output response does not attenuate until input frequencies exceed one cycle/20 minutes.

9. The adrenals have a secretory maximum of approximately 16 µg/min of cortisol in large dogs.

Urquhart and Li have described four models developed on an analog computer that simulate with varying degrees of success many of the qualitative and quantitative aspects of the above properties. In the present work we have adopted one of their models (model No. 2 [31]) and have rescaled its parameters and extended it slightly to include the static gain non-linearity.

Urquhart and Li have pointed out in their discussions of the aims of modeling of the adrenal response to ACTH that it is clearly desirable to use current knowledge or hypothesis about the mechanism of action of ACTH in the formulation of dynamic models of this subsystem. In such an effort properties of biochemical chains concerned with corticosteroidgenesis are used as constraining structure for the model. Their model helps to identify features of steroidogenesis and of ACTH action that are important in the dynamics of adrenocortical secretion.

The major pathway for the biosynthesis of cortisol from cholesterol includes at least eight reactions [24]:

Cholesterol: 20α-hydroxycholesterol: 20α, 22-dihydroxycholesterol: Δ^5-pregnenolone: Δ^5-pregnenedione: progesterone: 17α-hydroxyprogesterone: 17α-hydroxydeoxycorticosterone: cortisol.

Some branching into parallel sequences may occur. ACTH has a parametric action on the initial steps, and some negative feedback inhibition of the early reactions by intermediate products in the chains may be present. The cortisol secretory dynamic response of the adrenal gland to ACTH may be reproduced with 3', 5' adenosine monophosphate [32] and so the action of ACTH may involve the nucleotide as intermediate.

The model to be presented is based upon conservation of mass considerations in the above major pathway, and upon the kinetics of uni-molecular and bi-molecular reactions. Since production of one cortisol molecule requires modification of one cholesterol molecule, the steady-state relation between cortisol produced and cholesterol consumed (on a molar basis) is 1:1. We have arbitrarily, for the convenience of using the most familiar units for the secretory responses (µg/min), modeled the chain on a weight unit basis (i.e., the pools are given in µg) rather than on a molar basis. The input:output relation was maintained at 1:1 even though, because of the slight reduction in molecular weight as cortisol is created from cholesterol, the input:output mass relation should be 387:362. The small constant error from the molecular weight change can be corrected by addition of a scaling constant, but we did not include it since the specification of the mass of the pools in the chain is arbitrary. In the model, the eight-step major pathway has been abbreviated to a four-

F.E. YATES AND R.D. BRENNAN

step chain (Fig. 12) since at the present time quantitative biochemical information about in vivo corticosteroidogenesis is too meager to support more detailed modeling.

Each step in the pathway in Figure 12 is considered to be irreversible. The adrenocortical model assumes also that the major pathway involves two parallel pathways from cholesterol to hydroxylated cholesterol intermediates. One path (c-d) is forced in a parametric fashion by ACTH, and the other (c-c'-d) involves a coupled, bidirectional reaction that is catalyzed by a separate enzyme for the forward and back reactions. The back reaction is itself parametrically forced by the reactant, x, of another reaction that is also separately catalyzed for the forward and back directions. This latter back reaction is parametrically forced by ACTH. In addition, a source and a sink is present for reactant x.

The hierarchy of coupled and parametrically-forced reactions shown in Figure 12 is conjectural. The purpose of the model is to illustrate how the complicated dynamics and static properties of the adrenal cortex might arise from details of chemical kinetics. The quantitative biochemical study necessary to test the appropriateness of the specific reaction sequence of Figure 12 has not yet been technically possible. Until such quantitative biochemical work can be accomplished, simulations such as the one to be presented can serve as a guide toward possible biochemical mechanisms that can support the observed higher-level function. They can also rule out inappropriate biochemical models.

The complete set of equations for the model diagrammed in Figure 12 is given below:

Equations

Conservation of cholesterol in the pool immediately available for cortisol biosynthesis

9)

$$\frac{d(c)}{dt} = Q_{Ch} - k_1 c - k_2 c - (k_3 I) c$$

Delay

10)

$$I = c_{ACTH}.B(t - 2 \text{ mins})$$

Conservation equations for cascaded reactions in the main path

11)

$$\frac{d(d)}{dt} = k_2 c' + (k_3 I) c - k_5 d$$

MAMMALIAN ADRENAL GLUÇOCORTICOID SYSTEM

12)

$$\frac{d(e)}{dt} = k_5 d - k_6 e$$

13)

$$\frac{d(f)}{dt} = k_6 e - k_7 f$$

14)

$$\frac{d(g)}{dt} = k_7 f - k_{cs} g$$

Secretion of cortisol from its pool

15)

$$\dot{Q}_c = k_{cs} g$$

Coupling of blood flow to cortisol secretion

16)

$$k_3 = k_{bf3} V_{bf}$$

Parametric forcing function for the dissociation of xa

17)

$$\theta_{(I)} = pI + q$$

Conservation of reactant a

18)

$$\Sigma a = xa + a$$

19)

$$\frac{d(a)}{dt} = (\theta_{(I)} k_\beta) xa - k_\alpha(x)(a)$$

Parametric coupling of reactions involving a and b reactants

F.E. YATES AND R.D. BRENNAN

20)

$$\phi_{(x)} = mx - 1$$

Conservation of reactant b

21)

$$\Sigma b = c'b + b$$

22)

$$\frac{d(b)}{dt} = (\phi_{(x)} k_g) c'b - k_8(c') (b)$$

Conservation of reactant c'

23)

$$\frac{d(c')}{dt} = k_2 c + (\phi_{(x)} k_9) c'b - k_8(c') (b) - k_4 c'$$

Conservation of reactant x

24)

$$\frac{dx}{dt} = \dot{Q}_x + (\theta_{(I)} k_\beta) xa - k_\alpha(x) (a) - k_{x0}(x)$$

Limiting

25)

$$- a \gtrsim 10$$

26)

$$0.5 \lessgtr \phi_{(x)} \lessgtr 10$$

27)

$$\dot{Q}_c \lessgtr 16.5$$

Computer Simulation Diagram; Configuration Listing

The main sequence from cholesterol to cortisol is represented in Figure 13. Figure 14 specifies the tier of reactions that lead to parametric forcing of the parallel pathway from c to d, via c - c' - d. The complete adrenal model results

MAMMALIAN ADRENAL GLUCOCORTICOID SYSTEM

when the two programs are connected as shown in the Figures. The configuration of the complete adrenal model is given in Table IX.

Evaluation of Parameters from Data

The evaluation of the parameters of the adrenal equations is achieved as usual by adjusting their values until the model fits data from several independent experiments. Figure 15 shows the non-linear static gain characteristics of the model, compared to representative data from Urquhart and Li (from Figure 3 of Ref. 32). The effect of increased blood flow is illustrated.

Some of the dynamic characteristics of the model are shown in Figure 16, and are compared to data from Figure 2 and Figure 4 in Ref. 31, and Figure 6 from Ref. 32.

The complete list of parameter settings obtained from these experiments and others performed by Urquhart and Li are shown in Table X, with the initial conditions we used in the model subsystem when it was connected into the complete adrenal glucocorticoid system model.

Figure 17 shows other characteristics of the model subsystem that may be compared with similar results from several different analogous experiments reported by Urquhart and Li in Figure 3, from Ref. 31, and in Figures 5 and 7 from Ref. 32.

Figure 18 illustrates the use of the model to predict adrenocortical performance in experiments that are feasible, but that have not yet been performed in dogs in precisely the manner used during the experiments on the model.

SUBSYSTEM III: INPUT AND FEEDBACK CENTRAL ELEMENTS

Although data collection and modeling for the subsystems I and II described above are not easy, they are nevertheless rather straightforward in principal because the input and output for each subsystem are identifiable. Subsystem I accepts a cortisol secretion rate as input and produces a concentration of unbound cortisol in plasma as output; subsystem II accepts arterial blood concentration of ACTH as input and produces cortisol secretion rate as output. With respect to the central nervous system elements, however, the situation is different. Many different interoceptive and exteroceptive stimuli will provoke a response from the whole adrenal glucocorticoid system but the location and form of the immediate system inputs are not known. The output of the central elements, as we have lumped them for convenience in Figure 19, is ACTH secretion rate, which is a variable that is not yet accurately measurable under normal conditions of system operation.

F.E YATES AND R.D. BRENNAN

The relation between ACTH concentration in blood, and ACTH secretion rate was specified by assuming that ACTH is not bound in blood, that it is uniformly distributed into a volume of fluid (1 liter) somewhat larger than plasma volume (0.63 L), and that it is metabolized by a first-order clearance process, such that the half-life of ACTH in blood is 3.5 min. These specifications were based upon the work of Urquhart [29], and are in the ACTH DBM element of Figure 19.

The relationship between corticotropin releasing factor (CRF) secretion rate and ACTH secretion rate is not known in any species, so we have assumed a unity constant of proportionality as the simplest possible functional relationship. One of the purposes of modeling is the testing of such simplifying assumptions.

The series arrangement of the two feedback comparators with sign restrictions at their outputs has been justified in detail elsewhere [2,38]. That the system has multistage negative feedback now appears very likely [1,2,4], though the existence of a physiological negative feedback point at the anterior pituitary is still uncertain (dashed line in Figure 19). We did not include a pituitary feedback site in the configuration used for the experiments described in this paper. The comparators are simple algebraic summation devices that accept a positive input signal, a negative feedback signal, and then generate an error signal output restricted to zero or positive values. Of course the performance of the real neural elements may be more like a modulation, or some other operation, than like a subtraction, but in the absence of precise data we have again assumed the simplest functional relationship.

The equations describing the cascaded forward elements in Figure 19 are as follows:

Equations for Forward Elements

ACTH Distribution and Metabolism

28)

$$V_{ACTH} \frac{d(C_{ACTH.B})}{dt} = \dot{Q}_{ACTH} + \dot{Q}_{ACTH.i} - k_{ACTH} C_{ACTH.B}$$

ACTH Secretion Rate

29)

$$\dot{Q}_{ACTH} = k_{AP}(\dot{Q}_{CRF} + \dot{Q}_{CRF.i})$$

MAMMALIAN ADRENAL GLUCOCORTICOID SYSTEM

CRF Secretion Rate

30)

$$Q_{CRF} = k_{CRF} (y_{es} - y_m)$$

Comparator Equations

Median Eminence

31)

$$y_{em} = S_1 + S_b - y_{fb}$$

Septal Region

32)

$$y_{es} = S_2 + y_{em} - y_{fb} = S_b + s_1 + S_2 - 2y_{fb}$$

Negative Clipping

33)

$$(y_{es} - y_{em}), y_{es}, y_{em} \geqslant 0$$

The above algebraic details of the model, which are not state equations, may seem unrealistically simple, but in combination with the other better-documented features they serve as a useful starting point for deductions about the configuration of the inaccessible brain elements of this neuroendocrine system.

The Feedback Pathways

A current view about the adrenocortical negative feedback is that it operates slowly but effectively for low-level inputs of the system, but has little or no effect during the rapid responses to strong input signals ("stresses") [37]. The functional details of the feedback pathway are complex. The arrangement in Figure 19 shows that we have interpreted the experimental facts about the feedback pathway as indicating the presence of the following features:

1. The unbound cortisol concentration in plasma is the monitored, controlled variable [11].

2. The feedback path has a derivative-action, unidirectionally rate-sensitive component [3], such that when the rate of change of the plasma concentration of unbound cortisol exceeds a threshold level, an undelayed inhibitory feedback signal appears at the comparators. Evidence for the presence of a derivative component in the feedback path is shown in the left of Figure 20.

3. In parallel with the derivative action pathway is another feedback pathway that is not rate-sensitive, but which has a saturation property and a long delay. The evidence that the pathway reaches a saturation limit as corticosteroid levels in plasma are increased is based upon experiments with dexamethasone, in which it was shown that as the strength of a "stress" is increased, dexamethasone eventually fails to prevent an adrenocortical response [2]. Further increases in the dose of dexamethasone may then produce inhibition again, but a maximally effective dose of dexamethasone is ultimately clearly defined in such experiments, and larger doses have no further effect. From the studies with the computer model, it was discovered that a simple saturation function provides effective simulation of these results [38].

The evidence for the long delay has been obtained from the data at the right in Figure 20. This very long delay was surprising, and as noted previously, when it was included in this model scaled for the dog, it produced an oscillation after the initial conditions were applied (Figure 4). We attempted to simulate the results shown in Figure 20 other than with a pure delay of 120 minutes. However, the alternatives were not successful, and so we have left the delay in the model though it remains to be seen if it can be found in species other than the rat.

Feedback Equations

The feedback equations are:

Summation of Rate-Sensitive and Delayed Signals

MAMMALIAN ADRENAL GLUCOCORTICOID SYSTEM

34)

$$y_{fb} = n_4 y_{fr} + n_5 y_{fd}$$

Saturation and Delay Property of the Delayed Signal Pathway*

35)

$$y_{fd} = P_1 \left[1 - \varepsilon^{-P_2(C_{c.P} + C_{c.D})} \right]_{(t - 120 \text{ mins.})}$$

Rate-Sensitive Signal with Threshold. (The derivative signal is filtered slightly by a first-order lag.)

36)

$$y_{fr} = n_1 C_{c.P} - n_2 y - T$$

37)

$$dy/dt = n_3 (y_{fr})$$

Limiting

38)

$$y_{fd} \lessgtr P_1$$

Computer Simulation Diagram; Configuration Listing

The program configuration representing equations 28 through 38 is shown in Figure 21, and the complete configuration listing is given in Table XI.

---

*

The function in Equation (35) was simulated by use of the function generator element of the CSMP program.

F.E. YATES AND R.D. BRENNAN

Evaluation of Parameters

Since precise quantitative data are not available for the central elements of the adrenal glucocorticoid system, we have had to assign the parameter values by an indirect means. The technique is partially illustrated in Figure 22. The complete model was set up and a simulated standard step-infusion of ACTH for 20 minutes at 2 mU/min (40 mU total) was introduced. This infusion was found to produce a transient change in total plasma cortisol levels that peaked about half way up the physiological range for this variable, if the initial conditions had been established by setting S_b at 1.00 (when an input scaling factor of 5.00 was applied to element 51 in Figure 21). When a stress, S_1, of 1.00 was then also applied (again with an input scaling factor of 5.00 on element 51, Figure 21), the response matched exactly that produced by the ACTH infusion (Figure 22). Thus a one-unit step input as a "stress" S_1 on top of a basal, initial condition, S_b, produces in the model a step increase in ACTH release at the rate of 2 mU/min.

After the input levels were scaled with reference to ACTH release, the parameters of the delayed feedback path were adjusted to produce the data shown in Figure 23. These data simulate results previously published from analogous experiments performed in rats (Figure 1 of Ref. [2]. Final scaling for dogs is not yet possible until further experiments are done on this species.

The parameters of the rate-sensitive feedback path were adjusted to simulate the results described above by Figure 20. A corticosteroid constant infusion was simulated, and pulsed injections of ACTH (as specified in Figure 22) were given at the same time intervals as shown for the experiments in Figure 20. The simulation results are given in Figure 24. Then, under the same corticosteroid infusion conditions, a pulsed stress, exactly matched to the ACTH pulse (Figure 22), was given at the same intervals. Results are shown in Figure 25. Negative feedback inhibition of the stress response was complete at the first interval (30-50 minutes) (rate sensitive feedback effect) and also at the last interval (180-200 minutes) (delayed feedback effect). No inhibition was present at the middle interval (90-110 minutes). These results simulate exactly the experimental results shown in Figure 20, except that the time scale is appropriate for the simulated canine adrenal system, instead of the real rat adrenal system.

The listing of the parameter values and initial conditions for the central elements in subsystem III is given in Table XII.

MAMMALIAN ADRENAL GLUCOCORTICOID SYSTEM

THE COMPLETE MODEL FULLY SCALED

The fully-scaled complete model has been used in two different ways. First, the model is employed for verification of some properties of the adrenal glucocorticoid system that are known to exist, but that were not explicitly used in the modeling. For example, if a corticosteroid infusion is established, as in the real or simulated experiments of Figures 20, 24, and 25, and then discontinued before a test stress or an ACTH injection is applied, the ACTH will provoke the usual endogenous secretion of corticosteroid, but the stress response will nevertheless be inhibited (17). When the model was tested in this manner (Figures 26 and 27), the results were the same as those described above for the experimental animal, as the Figures demonstrate. Figure 28 shows another example of a result obtained with the model that is analogous to an experimental result not actually used in the development of the model [37].

Second, the model can be used to explore the functional properties of the adrenal glucocorticoid system under a very wide variety of experimental conditions not yet reproduced in the experimental laboratory, but nevertheless feasible. If the model makes accurate and nontrivial predicitions about the performance of the real system, then, of course, it will have clearly justified the efforts involved in its development. Such interacting prediction and testing between computer and dogs progresses slowly, but during the process the choice of experimental design in the laboratory is guided in a rational manner by the computer model, which embodies simultaneously and in a functional form many beliefs and observations about the whole adrenal glucocorticoid system. In no other way can so much knowledge and belief about this complex system be brought to bear upon experimental design. In that fact lies the true value of this model.

Leon Harmon once remarked with reference to neural modeling that he had noticed a direct relation between the degree of modesty with which an investigator presents his model, and the richness of the model in relevant properties. The models of the immodest tended to be most barren. Therefore, we emphasize that we know our model is a mere patchwork of data, theory and guesswork, based upon mixed results obtained from two different species. It lacks isomorphic properties because at every level of the model we have had to retreat from an attempt at isomorphic representation in the face of the so far insurmountable limitations of inadequate data. Yet we and others continue to be interested in this important system, without which vertebrate life is difficult or impossible to maintain. For those with that interest, the model stands as a comprehensive representation of many hypotheses about this neuroendocrine system. We shall be glad if it serves as a progenitor of a better model.

F.E. YATES AND R.D. BRENNAN

ACKNOWLEDGMENTS

We are indebted to Dr. John Urquhart for his data and model concerning the adrenocortical responses to corticotropin, which he generously supplied in advance of publication.

TABLE I   VARIABLES OF THE MODEL

		Symbol	Units
I.	**Concentrations**		
	1. Unbound plasma cortisol	$C_{c.P}$	ug/L
	2. Transcortin-bound cortisol in plasma	$C_{cT.P}$	ug/L
	3. Albumin-bound cortisol in plasma	$C_{cA.P}$	ug/L
	4. Total cortisol in plasma	$\Sigma C_{c.P}$	ug/L
	5. Total cortisol in virtual outer compartment 2	$C_{c.2}$	ug/L
	6. Unoccupied cortisol sites on transcortin	$C_{T.P}$	ug/L*
	7. Unoccupied cortisol sites on albumin	$C_{A.P}$	ug/L**
	8. Whole blood corticotropin (ACTH)	$C_{ACTH.B}$	mU/L
	9. Blood ACTH delayed 2 minutes	I	mU/L
II.	**Secretion Rates**		
	10. Cortisol	$\dot{Q}_c$	ug/min
	11. ACTH	$\dot{Q}_{ACTH}$	mU/min
	12. Corticotropin-releasing factor (CRF)	$\dot{Q}_{CRF}$	arbitrary mass/min
III.	**Pools of Metabolites Within Adrenal Gland**		
	13. Cholesterol	c	ug
	14. 20 α-hydroxycholesterol plus 20 α-22-dihydroxycholesterol	d	ug
	15. Δ^5 - pregnenolone + Δ^5 - pregnenedione + progesterone + 17 α- hydroxyprogesterone	e	ug
	16. 17 α - hydroxy - 11 - deoxycorticosterone	f	ug
	17. Cortisol	g	ug

The * indicates that the concentration of sites on transcortin is expressed in terms of cortisol equivalents, i.e., the increase in concentration of cortisol that would occur if the sites were filled with cortisol. The ** indicates that the concentration of the unoccupied cortisol sites on albumin was assumed to be so large as to be constant. This variable does not appear explicitly in the model, but was subsumed into the constant for the unimolecular adsorption reaction of albumin with cortisol described in Equation 7 of the text.

MAMMALIAN ADRENAL GLUCOCORTICOID SYSTEM

TABLE I   CONTINUED

18.	Cholesterol-derived precursors for components of pool d	c'	ug
19.	Complexing agent for precursor c'	b	ug
20.	Complexed c'	c'b	ug
21.	Reactant that shifts equilibrium for complexing of c' toward free c'	x	ug
22.	Complexing agent for reactant x	a	ug

III.	Pools of Metabolites Within Adrenal Gland	Symbol	Units
23.	Complexed reactant x	xa	ug

IV. *Neural Signals*

24.	Total feedback signal	y_{fb}	arbitrary units
25.	Delayed feedback signal	y_{fd}	" "
26.	Unidirectional, rate-sensitive feedback signal	y_{fr}	" "
27.	Error signal from septal comparator	y_{es}	" "
28.	Error signal from median eminence comparator	y_{em}	" "

TABLE II   NORMAL PARAMETERS OF THE MODEL SCALED FOR A 15 KG DOG.   THESE PARAMETERS WERE HELD CONSTANT DURING A GIVEN EXPERIMENT

	Parameter	Symbol	Normal Value
I.	*Distribution Volumes*		
1.	Cortisol inner compartment (plasma)	V_1	= 0.63 L
2.	Cortisol outer compartment	V_2	= 40 L*
3.	Distribution of ACTH as virtual single compartment	V_{ACTH}	= 1.0 L

---

*)   The volume of the outer compartment is larger than the body volume of the whole dog. This feature of two-compartment models for cortisol distribution, binding and metabolism has been noted also for humans [17]. This peculiarity of the outer compartment indicates that in the real system cortisol must be bound outside of the vascular system at concentrations higher in some regions than those that may exist in plasma. Even though the volume for the outer compartment is clearly a virtual volume, nevertheless it provides a satisfactory basis for simulation of the subsystem.

TABLE II   CONTINUED

Parameter	Symbol	Normal Value
II. *Total Amounts of Complexing Agents*		
4. Total plasma transcortin	$\Sigma C_{T.P}$	= 100 ug/Lt
5. Pool of complexing agent for reactant x	Σ_a	= 10 ug**
6. Pool of complexing agent for reactant c'	Σb	= 10 ug
III. *Constant Rates of Production or Flow*		
7. Cholesterol immediately available for cortisol biosynthesis	$\dot{Q}_{Ch}$	= 17.6 ug/min
8. Reactant x	$\dot{Q}_x$	= 0.20 ug/min
9. Blood flow to both adrenals	$\dot{V}_{bf}$	= 8 ml/min
IV. *Gains, Constant Multipliers, Scaling Terms*		
10. Sensitivity to x of rate coefficient for dissociation of c'b	m	30.0 = dimensionless
11. Threshold level of x required to force rate coefficient for dissociation of c'b	l	= 17.8 ug
12. Sensitivity to I of rate coefficient for dissociation of xa	p	= 0.046 L/mU
13. Basal residual value of forced component of rate coefficient for dissociation of xa, without forcing	q	= 0.035 dimensionless
14. Maximum (saturation) level for delayed feedback signal	P_1	= 10 dimensionless
15. Sensitivity of detector of unbound cortisol in delayed feedback path	P_2	= 0.1 dimensionless
16. Coupling coefficient between blood flow and steroid biogenesis	k_{bf3}	= 0.0016 $\frac{L}{mU \cdot ml}$
17. - 21. Gains in feedback pathways (arbitrary units)	n_1	= 100
	n_2	= 100
	n_3	= 0.01
	n_4	= 2.0
	n_5	= 1.0

**) The pool sizes for all reactants in the adrenal are arbitrarily given in μg units for convenience. However, since the model for corticosteroidogenesis is itself arbitrary, the pool sizes do not have absolute meaning.

†) The total transcortin concentration is given in cortisol equivalents, i.e., the concentration of transcortin-bound cortisol that would be present in plasma if all the cortisol binding sites on transcortin were filled.

MAMMALIAN ADRENAL GLUCOCORTICOID SYSTEM

TABLE II   CONTINUED

Parameter	Symbol	Normal Value
22. Coupling coefficient between CRF and ACTH secretion rates	k_{AP}	= 1.0 arbitrary units
23. Coupling coefficient between septal comparator output and CRF	k_{CRF}	= 1.0 arbitrary units

V. *Clearance Coefficients in ACTH and Cortisol Distribution, Binding Metabolism Elements*

24. Cortisol transfer from V_1 to V_2	k_{12}	= 1.12 L/min
25. Cortisol transfer from V_2 to V_1	k_{21}	= 1.12 "
26. Cortisol adsorption by albumin	k_{Aa}	= 0.12 "[††]
27. Cortisol release from albumin	k_{Ar}	= 0.075 "
28. Cortisol adsorption by transcortin	k_{Ta}	= 0.0015 L^2/ug min
29. Cortisol release from transcortin	k_{Tr}	= 0.026 L/min
30. Cortisol removed from body (liver, kidney, etc.)	k_{10}	= 0.63 L/min
31. Inactivation of ACTH	k_{ACTH}	= 0.20 L/min

VI. *Thresholds*

47. Threshold level for y_{fr}	T	arbitrary units

VII. *Rate Coefficients for Cortisol Biogenesis Processes:*

32. Cholesterol loss via processes not leading to cortisol	k_1	= 0.10 min^{-1}
33. Postulated conversion of cholesterol to precursor c'	k_2	= 0.005 min^{-1}
34. Conversion of c' to components in pool d	k_4	= 0.04 min^{-1}
35. Conversion of components of pool d to those of pool e	k_5	= 3.33 min^{-1}
36. Conversion of pool e to 17 α - hydroxy-deoxycorticosterone	k_6	= 3.33 min^{-1}

††)   The coefficient for adsorption of cortisol by albumin includes the variable $C_{A.P}$, as indicated in the footnote to Table I. This variable is assumed to be constant under the conditions of operation of the model, as described in [17].

TABLE II   CONTINUED

Parameter	Symbol	Normal Value

37. Conversion of 17 α - hydroxydeoxycorti-costerone into cortisol — k_7 = 3.33 min^{-1}

38. Association of c' with b — k_8 = 0.0025 ug^{-1}min^{-1}

39. Unforced component of rate coefficient for dissociation of c'b — k_9 = 0.0075 ug^{-1}min^{-1}

40. Association of x and a — k_α = 0.35 ug^{-1} min^{-1}

41. Unforced component of rate coefficient for dissolution of xa — k_β = 1.0 min^{-1}

42. Removal of reactant x — k_{xo} = 0.37 min^{-1}

43. Secretion of cortisol from its pool, g — k_{cs} = 1.0 min^{-1}

VIII. *Parametrically Forced Coefficients in Cortisol Biosynthesis*

44. ACTH input gain coefficient, blood flow coupled — k_3 = 0.013 min^{-1} mU^{-1}L normal blood flow

45. Rate coefficient for dissociation of c'b (Variable) — $(\phi_{(x)}k_9)$ min^{-1}

46. Rate coefficient for dissociation of xa (Variable) — $(\theta_{(I)}k_\beta)$ min^{-1}

TABLE III   PARAMETERS OF THE MODEL THAT DO NOT APPEAR IN THE SIMULATION DIAGRAMS OR PARAMETER VALUE LISTINGS.

Parameters from Table II	*Reason parameter is not shown in simulation diagrams and tabular listings for subsystems*
k_β	Unity value. Parameter is implicit
k_{AP}	"
k_{CRF}	"
k_{cs}	"
V_{ACTH}	"
P_1, P_2	Exponential function (Eq. #35) was simulated by function generator
k_{bf3}	This parameter is multiplied by adrenal blood flow to give parameter k_3 (Eq. #16). Parameter k_3 is used in model

MAMMALIAN ADRENAL GLUCOCORTICOID SYSTEM

TABLE IV   EXPERIMENTAL INPUTS AND PARAMETRIC FORCING FUNCTIONS.

A.   *Experimental Inputs of the Model (Constants or Variables)*

Input	Symbol	Units
Cortisol infusion or injection	$\dot{Q}_{c.i}$	ug/min
ACTH " " "	$\dot{Q}_{ACTH.i}$	mU/min
CRF " " "	$\dot{Q}_{CRF.i}$	arbitrary mass per min
Dexamethasone " "	C_{cD}	ug/L
Morphine " " "	$-y_m$	arbitrary units
Circadian basal level input	S_b	" "
Stress input #1, median eminence	S_1	" "
Stress input #2, septal region	S_2	" "
Adrenal blood flow	$\dot{V}_{bf}$	ml/min

B.   *Parametric Forcing Functions Within Adrenal Gland Subsystem*

Function	Units	Process Forced
$\theta_{(I)}$	dimensionless	dissociation of xa
$\phi_{(x)}$	ug	dissociation of c'b

TABLE V   BASAL CORTISOL SECRETION RATE (g/min) IN UNANESTHETIZED, UNILATERALLY
ADRENALECTOMIZED MALE DOGS.

Dog. No.	BW (kg)	(9:30AM) 0	20	40	60	80	100	120	140	160
1		0.17	0.14	0.02	0.10	0.08	0.24	0.21	0.22	0.64
	18.5									
1		0.17	0.11	0.17	0.13	0.11	0.11	0.08	0.08	0.07
2	23	0.37	0.37	0.25	0.28	0.28	0.28	0.25	0.37	0.80
3		0.35	0.52	1.4	0.67	1.1	3.5	1.1	6.9	0.86
	16									
3		0.36	0.68	1.1	0.82	0.36	0.62	0.44	0.62	0.57
4	19	0.18		8.0	0.76	0.37	0.85	0.13	0.19	----

1.0
hypophysect. ←————————→

TABLE VI

CONFIGURATION LISTING FOR CORTISOL DISTRIBUTION, BINDING AND METABOLISM SYSTEM.

*) The language symbols designating the element type are defined in Figure 1.

Output	Block No.	Type*	Input 1	Input 2	Input 3
$(C_{c.P})(C_{T.P})$	31	X	41	45	0
$V_1 \dfrac{d(C_{cT.P})}{dt} + V_1 \dfrac{d(C_{cA.P})}{dt} + V_2 \dfrac{d(C_{c.2})}{dt}$	32	+	47	48	49
$\Sigma C_{c.P}$	33	+	41	42	43
$C_{T.P}$	34	+	35	-42	0
$\Sigma C_{T.P}$	35	K	0	0	0
$\dot{Q}_{c.1}$	36	K	0	0	0
$C_{c.P}$	41	I	0	46	36
$C_{cT.P}$	42	I	0	47	0
$C_{cA.P}$	43	I	0	48	0
$C_{c.2}$	44	I	0	49	0
$C_{T.P}$	45	N	34	0	0
$V_1 \left[\dfrac{d(C_{c.P})}{dt} - \dot{Q}_{c.1} \right]$	46	W	25	32	41
$V_1 \dfrac{d(C_{cT.P})}{dt}$	47	W	31	42	0
$V_1 \dfrac{d(C_{cA.P})}{dt}$	48	W	41	43	0
$V_2 \dfrac{d(C_{c.2})}{dt}$	49	W	41	44	0

TABLE VII

INITIAL CONDITIONS (I.C.) AND PARAMETER SETTING FOR CORTISOL DISTRIBU-TION, BINDING AND METABOLISM SUBSYSTEM.

In this and other tables listing initial conditions, the inputs are all shown as zero (no forcing) except for the basal, circadian inputs S_b, which is shown (Table XII) at the level required to produce the initial conditions of the model illustrated in Figure 4.

| IC or Parameter | | | Block | IC or | | |
i	2	3	No.	Parameter 1	Parameter 2	Parameter 3
$\Sigma C_{T.P}$	—	—	35	100.0000	0.0000	0.0000
$\dot{Q}_{c.1}$	—	—	36	0.0000	0.0000	0.0000
IC	$1/V_1$	$1/V_1$	41	2.7535	1.5888	1.5888
IC	$1/V_1$	—	42	15.1788	1.5888	0.0000
IC	$1/V_1$	—	43	4.8608	1.5888	0.0000
IC	$1/V_2$	—	44	3.0085	0.0254	0.0000
unit gain	sign inversion	$-k_{10}$	46	1.0000	-1.0000	-0.6300
k_{Ta}	$-k_{Tr}$	—	47	0.0015	-0.0261	0.0000
k_{Aa}	$-k_{Ar}$	—	48	0.1200	-0.0748	0.0000
k_{12}	$-k_{21}$	—	49	1.1250	-1.1250	0.0000

TABLE VIII

RELATION OF THE TERMINAL, APPARENT HALF-LIFE FOR CORTISOL TO THE DOSE
OF CORTISOL ADMINISTERED, OR TO THE PRE-EXISTING TRANSCORTIN LEVELS, IN
STUDIES LIKE THOSE OF FIGURES 9 AND 10.

Dose of cortisol (mg)	Transcortin level (as ug/L of cortisol bound at saturation)	Terminal T 1/2 (mins)
0.28	100 (normal level)	73
3.6	100	87
36	100	96
0.28	100 (normal level)	73
0.28	200	78
0.28	500	88

MAMMALIAN ADRENAL GLUCOCORTICOID SYSTEM

TABLE IX

CONFIGURATION LISTING FOR ADRENAL CORTEX GLUCOCORTICOID SUBSYSTEM.

*) The language symbols designating the element types are defined in Figure 1.

Output	Block No.	Type*	Input 1	Input 2	Input 3
$(xa)(I)$	1	X	6	30	0
$-(x)(a)$	2	X	8	5	0
da/dt	3	W	6	1	2
$-a$	4	I	0	3	0
$-a$ (limited)	5	L	4	0	0
(xa)	6	0	5	0	0
$\dot{Q}_x$	7	K	0	0	0
x	8	I	7	3	8
mx	9	G	8	0	0
$\phi_{(x)}$	10	0	9	0	0
$\phi_{(x)}$ (limited)	11	L	10	0	0
$\phi_{(x)(c'b)}$	12	X	11	19	0
$(c')(b)$	13	X	15	17	0
db/dt	14	W	12	13	0
c'	15	I	16	14	15
k_2c	16	G	26	0	0
b	17	I	14	0	0
Σb	18	K	0	0	0
$c'b$	19	+	18	-17	0
$\dot{Q}_{Ch}$	20	K	0	0	0
d	21	I	27	15	21
e	22	I	0	21	22
f	23	I	0	22	23
g	24	I	0	23	25
$\dot{Q}_c$	25	L	24	0	0
c	26	I	20	29	26
k_3Ic	27	X	26	28	0
k_3I	28	G	30	0	0
$k_3Ic + k_2c$	29	+	27	16	0
I	30	4	59	0	0

F.E. YATES AND R.D. BRENNAN

TABLE X

INITIAL CONDITIONS AND PARAMETERS OF THE ADRENAL CORTEX GLUCOCORTICOID SUBSYSTEM.

IC or Parameter 1	2	3	Block No.	IC or Parameter 1	Parameter 2	Parameter 3
qk_β	pk_β	k_α	3	0.0350	0.0455	0.3500
IC sign inversion	---	---	4	-2.2652	-1.0000	0.0000
--- limit on -a	---	---	5	0.0000	-10.0000	0.0000
Σa	---	---	6	10.0000	0.0000	0.0000
$\dot{Q}_x$	---	---	7	0.2050	0.0000	0.0000
IC	unit gain	k_{xo}	8	0.4684	1.0000	-0.3740
m	---	---	9	30.0000	0.0000	0.0000
-1	---	---	10	-17.8000	0.0000	0.0000
upper & lower limit	$\phi_{(\overline{x})}$		11	10.0000	0.5000	0.0000
k_9	k_8	---	14	0.0075	-0.0025	0.0000
IC	unit gain	$-k_4$	15	18.3504	1.0000	-0.0400
k_2	---	---	16	0.0050	0.0000	0.0000
IC	---	---	17	31.3004	0.0000	0.0000
Σb	---	---	18	300.0000	0.0000	0.0000
$\dot{Q}_{Ch}$	---	---	20	17.6400	0.0000	0.0000
IC	k_4	$-k_5$	21	0.3419	0.0400	-3.3300
IC	k_5	$-k_6$	22	0.3509	3.3300	-3.3300
IC	k_6	$-k_7$	23	0.3605	3.3300	-3.3300
IC	k_7	$-k_{c3}$	24	1.3318	3.3300	-1.0000
max. $\dot{Q}_c$	---	---	25	16.5000	0.0000	0.0000
IC	unit gain	$-k_1$	26	158.4040	-1.0000	-0.1000
k_3	---	---	28	0.0130	0.0000	0.0000
IC 2 min ACTH delay	---	---	30	0.1825	2.0000	0.0000

MAMMALIAN ADRENAL GLUCOCORTICOID SYSTEM

TABLE XI

CONFIGURATION LISTING FOR THE CENTRAL ELEMENTS SUBSYSTEM.

*) The language symbols designating elements are defined in Figure 1.

Output	Block No.	Type*	Input 1	Input 2	Input 3
S_1	50	K	0	0	0
y_{em}	51	W	50	72	70
y_{em} (limited)	52	N	51	0	0
S_2	53	K	0	0	0
y_{es}	54	W	53	52	70
y_{es} (limited)	55	N	54	0	0
$y_{es} - y_m$	56	O	55	0	0
$\dot{Q}_{CRF}$	57	N	56	0	0
$\dot{Q}_{ACTH}$	58	O	57	0	0
$C_{ACTH.B}$	59	I	60	58	59
$\dot{Q}_{ACTH.i}/V_{ACTH}$	60	K	0	0	0
y_{fr}	61	W	41	62	0
y	62	I	0	61	0
y_{fr} with threshold	63	D	61	0	0
C_{cD}	64	K	0	0	0
$(C_{cD} + C_{c.P})$ Delayed 2 hours	65	l	41	64	0
y_{fd}	66	F	65	0	0
y_{fb}	70	W	63	66	0
S_b	72	K	0	0	0

TABLE XII

INITIAL CONDITIONS AND PARAMETER VALUES FOR CENTRAL ELEMENTS SUBSYSTEM.

*) This input establishes the baseline "resting" performance for the whole model.

1	IC or Parameter 2	3	Block No.	IC or Parameter 1	Parameter 2	Parameter 3
S_1	---	---	50	0.0000	0.0000	0.0000
Input scaling	Input scaling	sign inversion	51	5.0000	5.0000	-1.0000
S_2	---	---	53	0.0000	0.0000	0.0000
Input scaling	unit gain	sign inversion	54	5.0000	1.0000	-1.0000
$-y_m$	---	---	56	0.0000	0.0000	0.0000
$\dot{Q}_{CRF}$	---	---	58	0.0000	0.0000	0.0000
IC	$1/V_{ACTH}$	$-k_{ACTH}/V_{ACTH}$	59	0.2497	1.0000	-0.2000
Q_{ACTH}/V_{ACTH}	---	---	60	0.0000	0.0000	0.0000
n_1	n_2	---	61	100.0000	-100.0000	0.0000
IC	n_3	---	62	2.7535	0.0100	0.0000
Threshold for	y_{fr}	---	63	1.0000	-1000000.1264	0.0000
C_{cD}	---	---	64	0.0000	0.0000	0.0000
IC	120 min delay	---	65	2.7535	120.0000	0.0000
Upper limit of definition of arbitrary function		---	66	25.0000	0.0000	0.0000
n_4	n_5	---	70	2.0000	1.0000	0.0000
$S_b(IC)$*	---	---	72	1.0000	0.0000	0.0000

MAMMALIAN ADRENAL GLUCOCORTICOID SYSTEM

TABLE XII -- page 2

Settings for arbitrary function generator (piecewise linear approximation) for the function in equation 35. The numbers give the values of y_{fd} at ten equal finite increments in $(C_{c.P} + C_{cD})$ over the range of $(C_{c.P} + C_{cD})$ from zero to 25. y_{fd} changes linearly with $(C_{c.P} + C_{cD})$ between each pair of values.

Function Generator Specifications (Block 66)

0.0000	2.3030	4.0000	5.3000
6.7000	7.3000	7.8000	8.3000
8.7000	9.0000	9.2000	

F.E. YATES AND R.D. BRENNAN

REFERENCES

1. Chowers, I., S. Feldman and J.M. Davidson. Effects of intrahypothalamic crystalline steroids on acute ACTH secretion. Am. J. Physiol. 205:671, 1963.

2. Dallman, M.F. and F.E. Yates. Anatomical and functional mapping of central neural input and feedback pathways of the adrenocortical system. Mem. Soc. Endo., London, (in press).

3. Dallman, M.F., and F.E. Yates. Dynamic asymmetries in the corticosteroid feedback path and distribution-metabylism-binding elements of the adrenocortical system. Ann. N.Y. Acad. Sci. (in press).

4. Davidson, J.M. and S. Feldman. Cerebral involvement in the inhibition of ACTH secretion by hydrocortisone. Endocrinology 72:936, 1963.

5. Fortier, C. Nervous control of adrenocorticotrophic hormone secretion. In: The Pituitary Gland, Vol. 2 (G.W. Harris and B.T. Donovan, Eds.), Univ. of California Press, 1966.

6. Ganong, W.F. The central nervous system and the synthesis and release of adrenocorticotropic hormone. In: Advances in Neuroendocrinology (A.V. Nalbandov, Ed.) Urbana: Univ. of Illinois Press, 1963, 92.

7. Harwood, C.T. and J.W. Mason. Effects of intravenous infusion of autonomic agents on peripheral blood 17-hydroxycorticosteroid levels in the dog. Am. J. Physiol. 186:445, 1956.

8. Hume, D.M. and D.H. Nelson. Adrenal cortical function in surgical shock. Surg. Forum 5:568, 1955.

9. 1130 Continuous System Modeling Program (1130-CX-13X), Program Reference Manual, IBM Application Program H20-0282-0.

10. Jackson, W.S. Analog Computation. New York: McGraw-Hill, 1960.

11. Kawai, A and F.E. Yates. Interference with feedback inhibition of adrenocorticotrophin release by protein binding of corticosterone. Endocrinology 79: 1040, 1966.

12. Keller, N., L.R. Sendelbeck,U.I. Richardson, C. Moore and F.E. Yates. Protein binding of corticosteroids in undiluted rat plasma. Endocrinology 79:884, 1966.

13. Kuipers, F., R.S. Ely and V.C. Kelley. Metabolism of steroids: the removal of exogenous 17-hydroxycorticosterone from the peripheral circulation in dogs. Endocrinology 62:64, 1958.

14. Labrie, F. Interactions hormonales et rôle de la transcortine dans l'ajustement de l'active hypophyso-surrénalienne. (Ph.D. dissertation, Laboratoires d'Endocrinologie, Department de Physiologie, Faculte de Medicine, Universite Laval, Quebec), 1967.

15. Mangili, G., M. Motta, and L. Martini. Control of adrenocorticotropic hormone secretion. In: Neuroendocrinology, Vol. I (L. Martini and W.F. Ganong, Eds.), Academic Press, N.Y., 1966.

MAMMALIAN ADRENAL GLUCOCORTICOID SYSTEM

16. Mills, I.H., H.P. Schedl, P.S. Chen and F.C. Bartter. The effect of estrogen administration on the metabolism and protein binding of hydrocortisone. J. Clin. Endo. and Metabolism 20: 515, 1960.

17. Nugent, C.A., H.R. Warner, V.L. Estergreen and K.B. Eik-Nes. The distribution and disposal of cortisol in humans. Proc. Second Internat. Congr. Endocrinology (London). Excerpta Medica Internat. Congr. Series No. 83:257, 1964.

18. Peterson, R.E., J.B. Wyngaarden, S.L. Guerra, B.B. Brodie and J. Bunim. The physiological disposition and metabolic fate of hydrocortisone in man. J. Clin. Invest. 34:1779, 1955.

19. Peterson, R.E. and J.B. Wyngaarden. The miscible pool and turnover rate of hydrocortisone in man. J. Clin. Invest. 35:552, 1956.

20. Peterson, R.E. and C.E. Pierce. The metabolism of corticosterone in man. J. Clin. Invest. 39:741, 1960.

21. Steroid Dynamics (G. Pincus, T. Nakao and J.F. Tait, Eds.). Academic Press, N.Y., 1966.

22. Plager, J.E., G.A. Bray and J.E. Jackson. Pituitary-ACTH response to metopirone and endotoxin administration in the dog. Endocrinology 72: 876, 1963.

23. Riggs, D.S. The Mathematical Approach to Physiological Problems. Baltimore: Williams and Wilkins, 1963.

24. Samuels, L.T. and T. Uchikawa. Biosynthesis of adrenal steroids. In: The Adrenal Cortex (A. Eisenstein, Ed.), Boston: Little Brown and Company, 1967, p. 61.

25. Sayers, G. The adrenal cortex and homeostasis. Physiol. Rev. 30:241, 1950.

26. Tait, J.F. and S. Burstein. In vivo studies of steroid dynamics in man. In: The Hormones (G. Pincus, K. V. Thimann and E.B. Astwood, Eds.), Vol. V. Academic Press, N.Y., 1964, p. 441.

27. Thomasson, B. and R.W. Steenburg. Plasma clearance of cortisol and 11-deoxy cortisol in dogs. Am. J. Physiol. 208:84, 1965.

28. Urquhart, J., F.E. Yates and A.L. Herbst. Hepatic regulation of adrenal cortical function. Endocrinology 64:816, 1959.

29. Urquhart, J. Dynamics of ACTH in blood. Fed. Proc. 26:580, 1961 (Abstr.).

30. Urquhart, J. Adrenal blood flow and the adrenocortical response to corticotropin. Am. J. Physiol. 209:1162, 1965.

31. Urquhart, J. and C.C. Li. The dynamics of adrenocortical secretion. Am. J. Physiol. (in press).

32. Urquhart, J. and C.C. Li. Dynamic testing and modeling of adrenocortical secretory function. Ann. N.Y. Acad. Sci. (in press).

33. Yamamoto, W.S. and W.F. Raub. Models of the regulation of external respiration in mammals. Problems and promises. Computers and Biomed. Res. 1:65, 1967.

34. Yates, F.E., S.E. Leeman, D.W. Glenister and M.F. Dallman. Interaction between plasma corticosterone concentration and adrenocorticotropin-releasing stimuli in the rat: evidence for the reset of an endocrine feedback control. Endocrinology 69: 67, 1961.

35. Yates, F.E. and J. Urquhart. Control of plasma concentrations of adrenocortical hormones. Physiol. Rev. 42:359, 1962.

36. Yates, F.E. Contributions of the liver to steady-state performance and transient responses of the adrenal cortical system. Fed. Proc. 24, Pt. 1:723, 1965.

37. Yates, F.E. Physiological control of adrenal cortical hormone secretion. In: The Adrenal Cortex (A. Eisenstein, Ed.) Boston: Little Brown and Company, 1967, 133.

38. Yates, F.E., R.D. Brennan, J. Urquhart, M.F. Dallman, C.C. Li and W. Halpern. A continuous system model of adrenocortical function. In: The Systems Approach in Biology (M. Measarovic, Ed.), Springer-Verlag (in press).

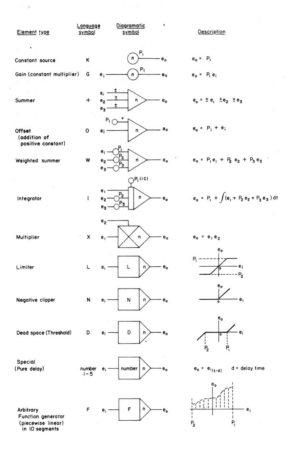

FIG. 1.   Designation of those functional elements from
the 1130 Continuous System Modeling Program that were
used in the adrenocortical system model.

The symbol n represents the block number assigned
for a specific use of the element.

F.E. YATES AND R.D. BRENNAN

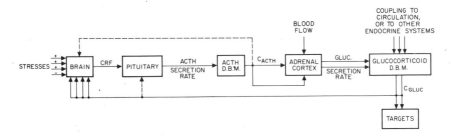

FIG. 2.   General organization of the adrenal glucocorticoid neuroendocrine system.

Abbreviations are: Adrenocorticotropic hormone (ACTH)
Corticotropin releasing factor (CRF)
Distribution–Binding–Metabolism Elements (D.B.M.)
Glucocorticoid hormones (GLUC)
Concentrations (C)

The system has multiple stimulatory, and possibly, inhibitory inputs, as well as multistage negative feedback. The system is coupled to other systems at several points.

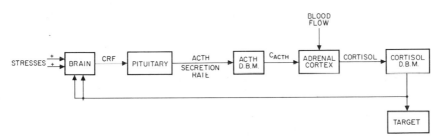

FIG. 3.   Diagram of the adrenal glucocorticoid system as modeled for a four-hour time domain.

Many of the features shown in Fig. 2 are not relevant in the performance of the glucocorticoid system over short time periods. The above figure shows the arrangement of the system that represents the configuration relevant for periods up to four hours. This reduced configuration served as the basis for the model.

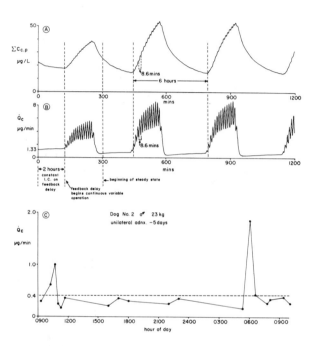

FIG. 4.   Baseline performance of the model under its initial
conditions, compared to the performance of the real system in
an unanesthetized dog.

The meaning of the symbols for the variables in
this and subsequent Figures is given in Table I.   The
data in part C of the Figure were obtained from a
dog that had been unilaterally adrenalectomized five
days prior to the experiment.   The adrenal secretion
rate shown for the remaining adrenal therefore represents the total secretion rate in the animal.   The
model has oscillatory behavior under its initial
conditions, because of a two-hour delay in the feedback pathway.

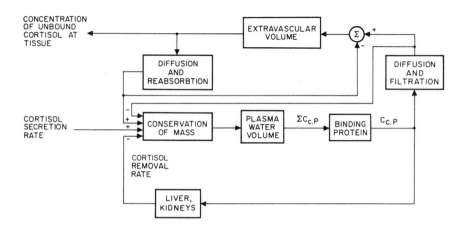

FIG. 5. Operational diagram for the cortisol distribution, binding and metabolism processes.

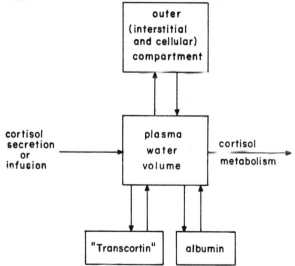

FIG. 6. Reduced diagram for the cortisol distribution, binding and metabolism processes.

The configuration shown in Fig. 5 is expressed in somewhat simpler form in the above Figure. This configuration served as the basis for the cortisol distribution, binding and metabolism subsystem of the model.

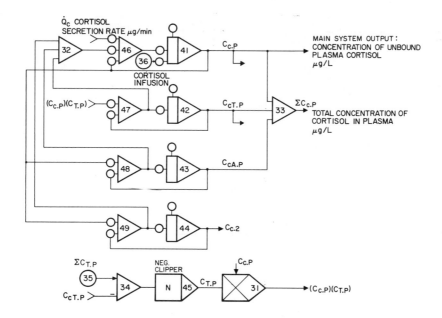

FIG. 7.   Simulation diagram representing the configuration shown in Fig. 6.
The symbols in this and subsequent simulation diagrams are defined
in Fig. 1.

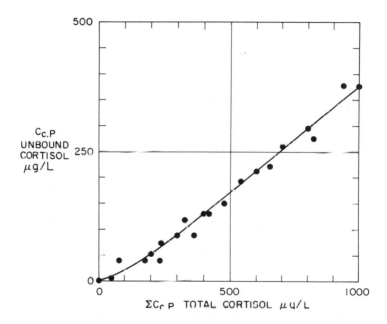

FIG. 8. Equilibrium protein-binding of cortisol in undiluted dog plasma
at 37°C.

The points represent experimental data, and the line represents
the computer fit of these data when the relevant parameters
of the program shown in Fig. 7 have been adjusted.

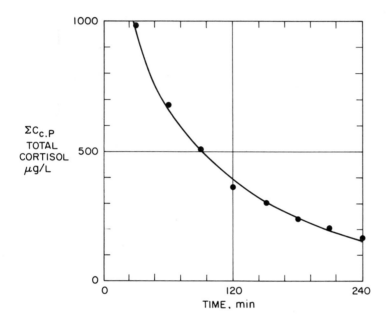

FIG. 9.   Disappearance of cortisol from plasma of adrenalectomized dogs,
following injection of 2 mg/kg i.v. at zero time.

The data points are taken from the work of Thomasson and
Steenberg [27]. The curve represents the computer fit of
the data after adjustment of the remaining parameters of the
model diagrammed in Fig. 7.

F.E. YATES AND R.D. BRENNAN

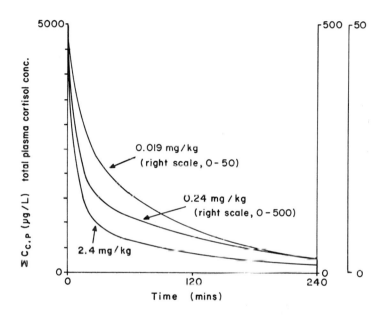

FIG. 10.   Non-linearity of the cortisol distribution, binding and metabolism subsystem of the model.

The fractional disappearance rate for cortisol depends upon the size of the injected dose in the model as in the real system. The curves shown were obtained from the model.

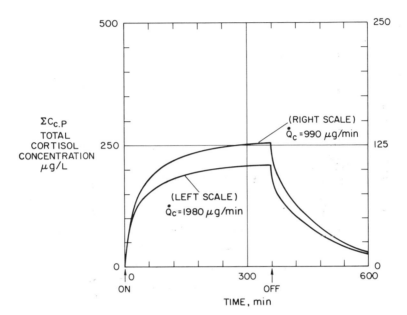

FIG. 11.   Other evidence for non-linearity in the cortisol distribution, binding and metabolism process.

The curves shown were obtained from the cortisol distribution, binding and metabolism subsystem of the model. When a steady infusion of cortisol is turned on, the plasma cortisol concentration rises smoothly toward a steady-state plateau level. If the infusion rate is doubled, the new steady-state plateau level is less than twice the previous value. Thus, this subsystem does not obey the Superposition Principle. These non-linearities of the distribution, binding, and metabolism processes have been observed in the real adrenal glucocorticoid system [3,17].

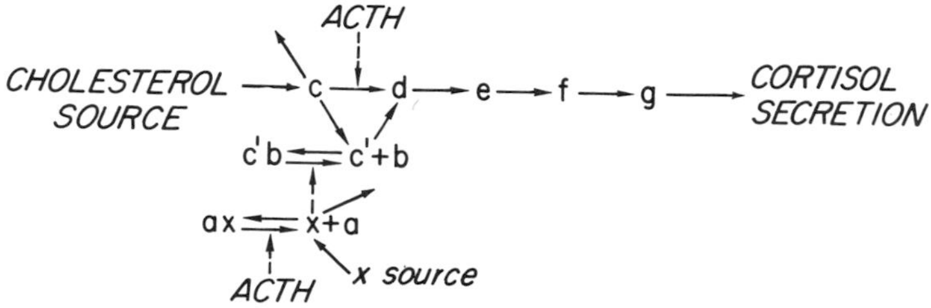

F.E. YATES AND R.D. BRENNAN

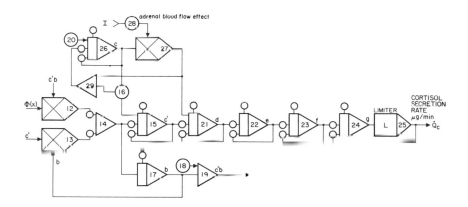

FIG. 12.   Kinetic model for the biosynthesis of cortisol in the adrenal cortex.

    This model postulates a tier and cascade of reactions capable of generating the dynamic properties of the adrenal cortex.

FIG. 13.   Simulation diagram for the cascaded reactions of Fig. 12 for the conversion of cholesterol to cortisol.

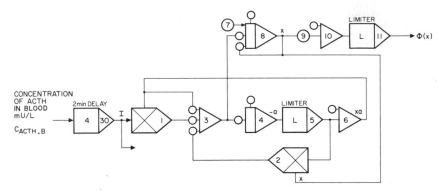

FIG. 14.   Simulation diagram for the tier of reactions in Fig. 12 that parametrically force the cascade modeled as in Fig. 13.

The diagrams of Figs. 13 and 14 together comprise the complete adrenocortical subsystem model.

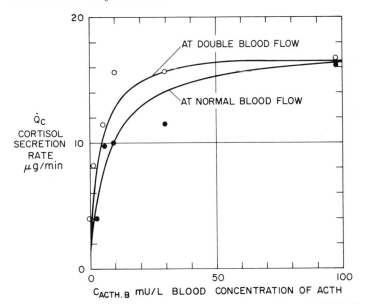

FIG. 15.   Non-linear, static gain characteristics of the dog adrenal.

The data points are from the work of Urquhart and Li [30,32]. The curves represent the computer fit of the data.   In the experiments and in the simulation, transients were allowed to die out and only steady-state levels were recorded after blood concentration of ACTH was changed.

F.E. YATES AND R.D. BRENNAN

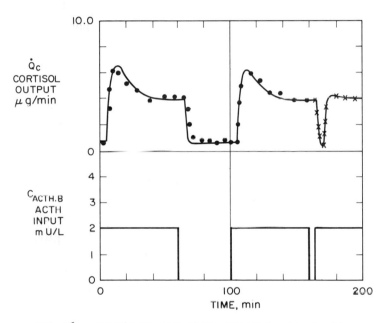

FIG. 16. Dynamic response of the adrenal to step forcing.

The data (closed circles and crosses) are from two different experiments performed by Urquhart [31,32]. The curves represent the performance of the computer adrenocortical subsystem model.

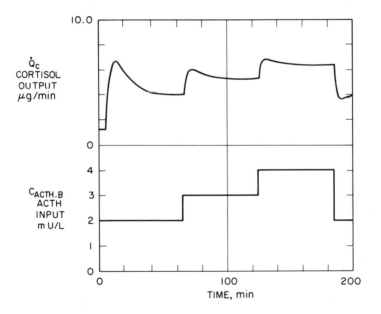

FIG. 17.   Response of the model adrenocortical subsystem to
successive step increases in ACTH.

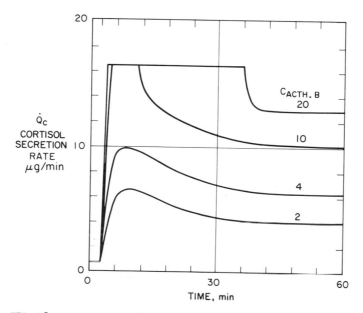

FIG. 18.   Response of the adrenocortical subsystem to ACTH step infusions of various magnitudes, turned on at zero time.

The ACTH inputs produced step increments in blood concentrations of ACTH, ranging from 2 to 20 mU/L as indicated.

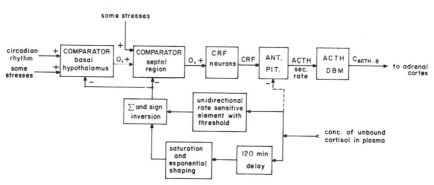

FIG. 19.   Operational diagram of the central elements of the adrenal glucocorticoid neuroendocrine system.

Cascaded forward elements, and parallel feedback pathway elements are shown.

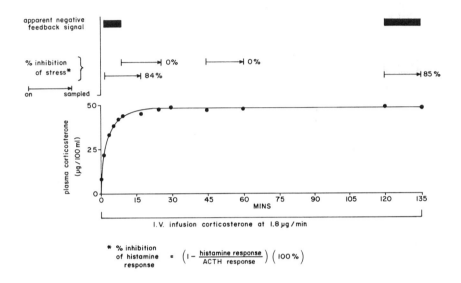

FIG. 20.   Experimental results from studies on rats indicating the
existence of a rate-sensitive component and a parallel two-hour delay
component in the feedback pathways.

A steady infusion of cortisterone was used to elevate plasma
corticosterone levels to about half the physiological maximum.
ACTH was given as a pulse injection (several seconds) at various
indicated times ("on") during the corticosterone infusion, to
calibrate the system for the summation of endogenous plus
exogenous corticosteroid inputs. The response was measured 15
minutes later ("sampled"). Then a pulsed stress was applied
in separate experiments, at the same times relative to the
infusion as were used for the ACTH. The system output was
expressed as a percent inhibition of the stress response,
defined as indicated at the bottom of the Figure. These
experiments have been given in detail elsewhere [3].

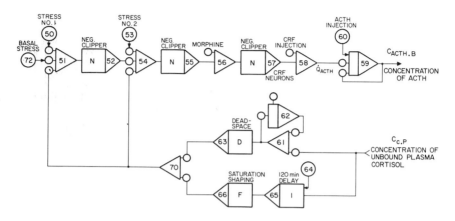

FIG. 21. Simulation diagram for the central elements subsystem of the model.

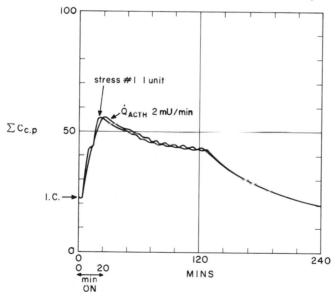

FIG. 22. Calibration of a stress input according to ACTH released.

A step infusion of ACTH was turned on for 20 minutes. Similarly, a step stress was applied to the complete model, so the response matched that obtained with the ACTH. This level of stress was defined as one unit, and produced ACTH release at the rate of 2 mU/min in the complete model.

MAMMALIAN ADRENAL GLUCOCORTICOID SYSTEM

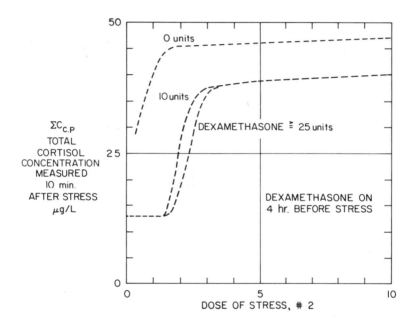

FIG. 23. Effect of increasing doses of dexamethasone on the response of the complete model to graded input signals.

The steady dexamethasone signal was initiated four hours before the stress input signal was turned on for 10 minutes. Therefore the properties demonstrated in this Figure apply to the delayed feedback pathway. These results are similar to those obtained from animal experiments [2]. The units for the doses of dexamethasone are arbitrary.

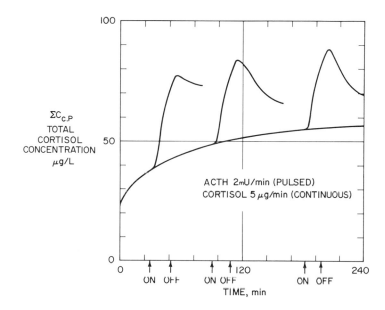

FIG. 24.   Results obtained in the complete model when rectangular pulses
of ACTH infusions, at three different time periods, are superimposed
upon a steady infusion of cortisol.

The endogenous cortisol released by the ACTH, and the exogenous
cortisol infused add to produce the three peaks shown. The
continuous smooth curve represents the results obtained with
the cortisol infusion alone. The three pulses of ACTH were
given in separate experiments, and are not given sequentially
in the same experiment.

MAMMALIAN ADRENAL GLUCOCORTICOID SYSTEM

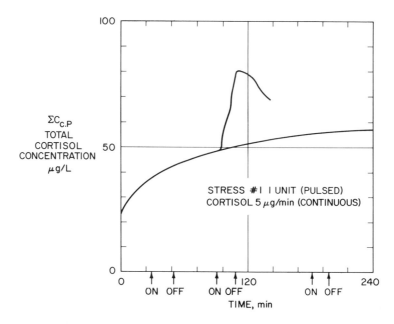

FIG. 25.   Demonstration of rate-sensitivity and two-hour delay in parallel feedback pathways of the model.

The lower, continuous smooth curve represents the result in the complete model following a step infusion of cortisol. In separate experiments, at three different time intervals, a unit stress was applied as a rectangular pulse for 20 minutes. Endogenous ACTH and cortisol release were completely prevented at the early application of the stress, when cortisol levels were rising (derivative feedback action), and after the infusion had been continued for more than two hours (delayed feedback action). In contrast, if the stress was applied after the rapid rate of rise of plasma cortisol levels was over, but before the two-hour delay was over, then the stress was effective in provoking endogenous ACTH and cortisol release which added to the cortisol levels produced by the infusion of exogenous cortisol. The simulation results shown in Figures 24 and 25 are analogous to those obtained from animal experiments shown in Figure 20.

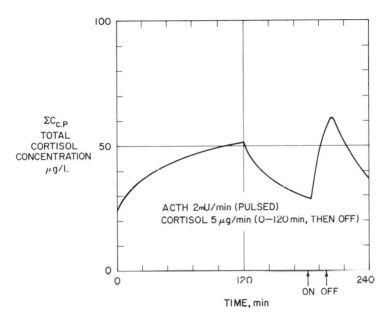

FIG. 26.   Demonstration that the late inhibition of the system
produced by elevation of plasma corticosteroid levels, as shown in
Figure 20, represents a delay rather than a lag or integral feedback action.

In the complete model a step infusion of cortisol
was maintained for 120 minutes, and then removed.
Plasma cortisol levels then began to drop, until
endogenous cortisol was released following a 20-
minute rectangular pulse of ACTH given later. The
endogenous cortisol produced following ACTH added
on to the falling levels of exogenous cortisol.
These results served as a control for the experiment
shown in Fig. 27.

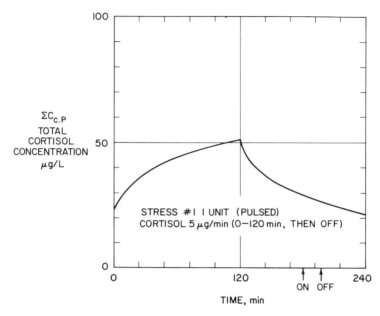

FIG. 27.   Evidence for delay rather than lag or integral action in
the feedback path.

When the experiment shown in Fig. 26 was repeated with
a unit stress substituted for the rectangular pulse
of ACTH, endogenous release of ACTH and cortisol was
completely inhibited by the prior infusion of cortisol
even though the infusion had been discontinued and
plasma cortisol levels were declining. This result
is exactly the same as the shown in the right of Fig. 25,
so neither a lag nor an integral action characterize
the feedback path, since either of these features
would produce less inhibition under the conditions
shown above, than under the conditions shown in Fig. 25.
These results were expected of the model, of course,
since a delay had been built into the feedback path.
They are shown to emphasize that a delay provides the
same properties as had been discovered in experiments
on animals done under analogous conditions [3].

F.E. YATES AND R.D. BRENNAN

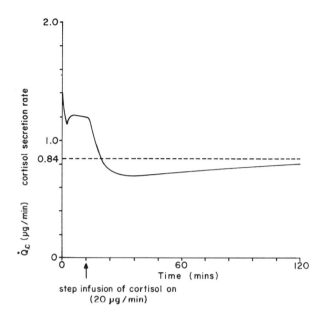

FIG. 28.   Effect of a step infusion of cortisol at a high level, on the basal secretion of cortisol (initial conditions) in the model.

The initial brief transient change in cortisol secretion rate when the model is turned on, before the cortisol infusion is begun, occurs because the various initial conditions throughout the model were not perfectly matched. This transient is an artifact. The initial secretion rate is given by the plateau level of about 1.2 µg/min. The endogenous secretion of cortisol ceases almost immediately after the exogenous cortisol infusion is begun (derivative feedback action). The dashed line represents the level of steady-state residual secretion of cortisol from the adrenal gland in the model when there is no ACTH input (simulated hypophysectomized animal). The secretion rate transiently undershoots the zero-input level as a result of the properties inherent in the model of the adrenal cortical subsystem. The residual secretion in hypophysectomized animals in this model is at the upper limit of the levels observed in animals, which range from less than 0.1 up to the level shown.

3. GLUCOSE HOMEOSTASIS: A BRIEF REVIEW

G.F. CAHILL, JR.[**], and J.S. SOELDNER
Department of Medicine, Elliott P. Joslin Research Laboratory, Harvard Medical School and Peter Bent Brigham Hospital, and the Diabetes Foundation, Inc., Boston, Mass.

INTRODUCTION

This presentation will separate glucose homeostasis into several distinct physiological entities. One is concerned with the maintenance of a constant glucose level during times when calories are not available from the environment. Another is concerned with the perturbation when an external supply of calories, glucose in particular, is made available from the environment. For simplicity, these will be referred to as the "fasted" and "fed" states, respectively. Three abnormal states will also be discussed. One is a "super-fasted" state whereby, with or without external calories, only the fasted signal is in operation. Another is the "inappropriate fed" state whereby the fed signal is operative in spite of an absence of externally derived calories. Finally, the third, the "fasted-adapted" state, occurs only after a prolonged period of starvation.

FASTED STATE

In order to study man in as near to a steady state as possible, subjects must be fasted for over a week. This period of time is chosen, since for the first four or five days of fasting there is a rise and fall in nitrogen excretion in addition

---

[*] Supported in part by grants from the U.S. Public Health Service (AM-09584, AM-09748, AM-05077, and 8 M01-FR-31-05, and the John A. Hartford Foundation, New York, N.Y.).

[**] Investigator, Howard Hughes Medical Institute.

G.F. CAHILL, JR., AND J.S. SOELDNER

to probable readjustments in glycogen levels. From the sixth day on, there is a progressive but gradual decrease in nitrogen excretion over the next few weeks, when a minimum of 3 to 4 grams/day is achieved. This phenomenon is best seen as the contribution of protein to total calorie expenditure as shown in Figure 1 which is taken from Benedict's classical study published fiftythree years ago [1]. Blood glucose and serum insulin concentrations in six of our subjects fasted for seven and a half days are presented in Figures 2 and 3; and, in Figure 4, correlations between these two are plotted for each day for each subject. The concentration of glucose (plotted the y axis) is related to insulin concentration (plotted on the x axis) by the equation y = 57.2 + 1.22 x, suggesting a close physiological relationship between glucose concentration and insulin concentration [2]. The bulk of this paper will be directed to further elaboration and understanding of this relationship.

The first question to be asked is whether, in the prolonged fasted state, the effect of insulin is to alter inflow (gluconeogenesis) or to accelerate outflow (glucose assimilation), either or both processes being capable of maintaining the constant glucose concentration noted in Figure 2. Good evidence that the control is exerted on the inflow mechanism is derived from two facts. The first is that man possesses only 200 grams of carbohydrate reserve, and for a prolonged fast he must synthesize glucose mainly from protein to satisfy the needs of the central nervous system. In order to survive this prolonged fast, particularly in a primitive setting, glucose consumption must be markedly diminished to conserve body protein; and it is a far more economical process to regulate glucose concentration by regulating its inflow as opposed to altering its outflow. The second piece of evidence is that, if one administers a glucose load, the body fails to recognize the load for a period of an hour or so. The decrease in glucose concentration as seen in Figure 5 is primarily a function of glucose loss in the urine, and therefore not due to any alteration in peripheral glucose assimilation [2]. Thus, the glucose removal rate in man fasted for several days appears to be relatively slow and fixed, corroborating the statement that inflow must be the fine regulatory control mechanism in glucose homeostasis. That this inability to metabolize glucose is not due solely to decreased insulin release is shown in Figure 6. A rapid increase in insulin does occur after the glucose load in both the brief fasted state (overnight fast) or in the prolonged fasted state (seven and a half days), but the insulin response in the latter is markedly attenuated. Again, this inability to alter glucose removal rate strongly supports the conjecture that the fine regulation of glucose concentration is due to fine adjustments in the rate of inflow and cannot be due to any alteration in outflow.

GLUCOSE HOMEOSTASIS

Glucose inflow is a function of two organ systems which, by and large, operate relatively independently of each other. Liver is by far the most important in this respect, but under certain circumstances kidney may be the more important site of gluconeogenesis. Many studies have been directed to locating the hormonal control of hepatic gluconeogenesis, and much argument has been devoted to the question of whether or not insulin alters this process, and, if so, by what mechanism and at what step or steps [23]. Numerous enzymatic reactions in liver have been shown to be altered by hormonal administrations or deficits; but, currently, more and more investigators are turning to the hypothesis that the primary fine control of the gluconeogenic rate is accomplished by variation in substrate presentation [6,11]. In other words, the rate of gluconeogenesis is directly proportional to the concentration of the gluconeogenic precursors. The changes in enzyme activities by hormonal alterations, therefore, merely set the gross limits of the maximum and minimum rates for saturating concentrations of substrate. Further evidence for this view is supplied by the fact that hormonally induced alterations usually occur over a period of several hours; whereas, the rate of gluconeogenesis is altered within seconds after a change in substrate concentration.

Another more interesting phenomenon is that free fatty acids, by providing for liver's own energy needs [11,22], and not as a direct substrate for gluconeogenesis, displaces potential glucose precursors (namely, amino acids) from oxidation into glucose synthesis. Thus, for any given concentration of glucose precursor, an increase in free fatty acid level increases its incorporation into glucose by preventing its oxidation to CO_2.

The aforementioned facts suggest, therefore, that the control of "steady state" glucose concentrations in blood lies outside the liver and is a function of insulin, with insulin possibly working directly on peripheral tissues and regulating rates of precursor release. Adipose tissue, the source of free fatty acids, is extremely sensitive to the effects of insulin. An overall scheme for its metabolism is presented in Figure 7. In the presence of high concentrations of insulin, glucose uptake by tissues is stimulated, fatty acids are synthesized from the glucose, made into triglyceride and stored. In addition, lipolysis is also inhibited by insulin and free fatty acids are not released. With low insulin concentrations, glucose uptake ceases, triglyceride is hydrolyzed to free fatty acids and glycerol, and these moieties are released into the blood stream. Thus, the overall scheme can be summarized as in Figure 8. The precise point where free fatty acid release and glucose uptake are at 0 is not known, but probably approximates 5 μUnits/ml of insulin. It is certain that fatty acid release is inhibited with insulin concentrations well below this very low concentration. It should be emphasized to the non-biologist that insulin is here exerting a metabolic effect at 10^{-11} molar concentrations.

Turning to amino acids, insulin has been shown to exert a significant metabolic effect in increasing amino acid incorporation into muscle protein at concentrations of 50 µUnits/ml [13]. No studies have been directed to see how much greater is this tissue's sensitivity in vivo; however, other in vivo studies in man have shown a significant reduction in plasma alpha amino nitrogen at levels of endogenous insulin below 50 µUnits/ml [4]. The insulin effect, as schematically shown in Figure 9, is either at amino acid entry into the tissue or else on the protein-synthetic mechanism inside the tissue. There is evidence for both. In the absence of insulin, and in the presence of adrenal glucocorticoid, muscle protein is hydrolyzed and free amino acids are released.

In summary, therefore, the insulin effect appears to be as shown in Figure 10, whereby a feedback loop is composed of both substrates and hormones. From the Figure, it is easy to conclude by extrapolation that an inappropriate overproduction of insulin, the "inappropriate fed" state, would result in a decrease in plasma free fatty acid (FFA) and amino acid (AA) levels, diminished gluconeogenesis, hypoglycemia, and ultimately death. Conversely, in the "super-fasted" state, a marked decrease or absence in insulin concentration would result in excessive FFA and AA mobilization, excessive gluconeogenesis, a marked increase in glucose concentration with loss into the urine, and as stated by Areteus over two millenia ago, the "flesh melteth down into urine," the classical description of uncontrolled diabetes.

As stated before, kidney is also capable of gluconeogenesis, and recent experiments have shown that the deaminated and deamidated residues of amino and amido acids are incorporated into glucose. Thus, glucose production is coupled to ammonia production, being increased in states of acidosis and decreased in states of alkalosis, as shown in Figure 11 [9, 12].

HOW FINE IS GLUCOSE REGULATION?

Returning to liver, the enzymes involved in the inflow and outflow of glucose are illustrated in Figure 12. Studies to be presented later in this paper will show that normal man is sensitive to changes in glucose concentration of at least 5 mg%, as evidenced by altered concentrations of insulin. By standard enzyme kinetics, it seems highly improbable that enzyme levels per se (by the nature of the velocity of the reaction being a function of the logarithm of the substrate concentration) could be regulated with such fine adjustment, even if insulin could acutely alter the levels of these enzymes, which it apparently does not. Thus, again, the evidence is strongly in favor of the beta cell and its insulin release being the fine adjustment for glucose concentration, doing so by controlling peripheral release of substrate, which, as described above, is capable of altering the rate of gluconeogenesis within seconds.

QUANTIFICATION

Previously we have described the qualitative events governing substrate release and gluconeogenesis. This section will now deal with the amount of substrate flowing from tissue to tissue per unit time. By classical indirect calorimetry, a normal 70 kg man, basal, utilizes about 1800 calories/day. In Figure 13, is summarized the amount of substrate metabolized over a 24-hour period. As can be seen, glucose output by liver approximates 180 grams, of which 144 grams are terminally oxidized to CO_2 by nerve (mainly brain) and 36 grams are metabolized by glycolytic tissues to lactate and pyruvate. Of the glycolytic tissues, the red cells and white cells account for the bulk of this metabolic moiety. Also seen is the fact that one fourth of the free fatty acid flux is removed by liver, which, when partially oxidized to ketones, provides the necessary energy for liver function. The remainder of the carcass utilizes these ketones, in addition to the other three fourths of the fatty acid flux. Lastly, tallying up the available gluconeogenic precursors, 16 grams of glycerol plus 36 grams of lactate and pyruvate plus 75 grams of amino acids are inadequate to provide 180 grams of glucose, the difference being made up by minimal hepatic glycogenolysis.

In Figure 14 is shown the "super-fasted" state in which there is no check on the release of peripheral fuels due to a relative or absolute lack of insulin. Gluconeogenesis and ketogenesis increase, and both substrates spill in the urine. The ketones (really β-hydroxybutyric and acetoacetic acids), being strong acids, are excreted with sodium and potassium; and therefore life is threatened by acidosis and hypovolemia should the condition persist for more than a day or so. It should be emphasized that these numbers are estimates derived from the literature plus some actual determinations made in our laboratory [2, 17].

Finally, as mentioned earlier, nitrogen excretion with more prolonged starvation continues to decrease until a minimum of 3 to 4 grams/day is achieved. The amount of glucose synthesized from this minimal amount of protein, even when added to the amount of precursor returning to the liver as lactate and pyruvate and added to the amount capable of being synthesized from glycerol, is yet inadequate to provide ample glucose for brain. This problem is solved by brain adapting to utilization of ketoacids, as shown in Figures 15 and 16 [17]. In other words, even brain has adapted to fat utilization, but by the devious method of utilizing a product of partial fat oxidation.

G.F. CAHILL, JR., AND J.S. SOELDNER

THE FED STATE

It is obvious that this well-balanced hormone-fuel interrelationship is periodically perturbed by a variety of fuel or fuel precursors entering the system. Due to the vast heterogeneity of these fuels (meals) containing carbohydrate, protein, and fat, and the huge variations in quantity that are successfully assimilated at regular or irregular intervals by animals and man, it is impossible to do more than generalize concerning the gross changes that take place in the prime fuels (glucose, free fatty acids, and amino acids) and in the hormones (insulin, glucagon, growth hormone, etc.) that may be altered as a function of fuel input. The fed state is also immensely complicated not only by the necessities to pass this fuel mixture in a raw state into a digestive system (which is really external to the utilizing system) but also by the variability in the rates of transferral of these fuels into the circulation. Finally, there is evidence that factors other than the fuels (mainly glucose and amino acids) may synergize insulin release over and above that of the fuels themselves [7, 15, 19].

Therefore, there is insufficient quantitative data available to apply to the physiological fed state, especially in the area of the interaction of insulin with other hormones or gastrointestinal factors stimulating insulin secretion [5]. In order to obtain utilizable data, it has been necessary to produce a most unphysiologic situation in that a specific fuel, glucose (rarely found in a pure state as a natural food), is introduced directly into the system (by peripheral vein) during an extremely short period of time (three minutes). The influence of this model perturbation upon concentrations of blood glucose (BG), serum insulin (IRI), and plasma free fatty acids (FFA) is shown in Figures 17 and 18. The levels were obtained in 11 normal healthy male volunteers and in 5 other healthy males who are the offspring of two documented diabetic parents (prediabetics). A wide variety of tests specifically designed to reveal a defect in glucose utilization were performed upon the prediabetics; however, no evidence was found of any blood glucose defect during any of the tests. It is generally accepted that these prediabetics have up to 100 percent probability of eventually developing at least mild diabetes. It can be seen that the load of glucose (0.5 gm per kg body weight) produces a maximal rise in blood glucose one minute after the termination of the infusion which subsequently falls according to what appears to fit a first order equation [8]. The rate of disappearance of the blood glucose levels has been calculated for each test during the ten to sixty-minute interval, and the mean rates (K - percent per minute disappearance) are shown in Table 1. Similar to blood glucose levels, the maximal levels of serum IRI are seen at the one-minute interval, and these fall until baseline levels are reached at the 120-minute interval. Levels of plasma free fatty acids fall rapidly after the glucose load and reach a nadir sixty minutes after the infusion.

Further studies in normal healthy subjects (100+) confirmed that following an overnight fast, a rapid intravenous glucose load generated maximal elevations in serum IRI one minute after the termination of the infusion in approximately 95 percent of instances.

In a smaller number of healthy controls, further studies have shown that not only glucose infusions, but also tolbutamide infusions (a sulfonylurea compound widely used in treatment of mild diabetes), can produce significant rises of serum insulin in a peripheral vein within 120 seconds following the initiation of the infusion. Making various estimates of circulation times (viz., glucose to pancreas, and insulin to arm vein), it appears that beta cells respond to glucose with a relatively large secretion of insulin that occurs within thirty seconds after the arrival of the glucose in the pancreas (Figure 19). Studies performed in the portal vein of rats (Figure 20) demonstrate this rapid insulin release as have studies of the isolated pancreas by Grodsky et al. [10].

This evidence is highly suggestive of the importance of insulin as a prime regulator of glucose uptake by tissues (the rapid disappearance rate of the blood glucose following the load) and a major suppressor of lipolysis in adipose tissue (fall in FFA). Numerous studies of the effect of intravenous insulin administration upon BG and plasma FFA have shown that the plasma FFA fall is a function almost exclusively of the insulin levels.

Furthermore, the relative levels of BG and IRI during the test have suggested that not only does the glucose load evoke a rapid outpouring of insulin from the beta cell, but that the ambient levels of serum IRI are related to the ambient levels of BG. To examine the relationship between IRI and BG, further studies were done examining the levels of both IRI and BG in the same blood samples taken every two minutes following the end of the glucose infusion for a period of 120 minutes. Figures 21 and 22 depict two such studies, and it can be seen that an extremely high correlation exists between IRI and BG. The relative excess IRI in relation to BG during the first ten to twelve minutes following the glucose load has been shown to be due to the slower diffusion rate of insulin from the vascular to extravascular compartment when compared to glucose [18]. Analysis of over 100 rapid intravenous glucose tests in normal subjects has indicated that a statistically significant correlation exists between these two moieties in approximately 95 percent of tests. Therefore, for descriptive and comparative purposes, it has been possible to express the serum IRI-BG changes during this type of glucose loading as a linear regression equation quantifying the relationship as the slope constant (b) of the equation $y = a + bx$, where IRI = y, BG = x, a = constant.

G.F. CAHILL, JR., AND J.S. SOELDNER

Further studies have been done examining this relationship during a second type of glucose-loaded state; namely, following the administration of 100 gms of glucose by mouth. As stated in the outset, a greater number of unknown variables are operative following oral administration (absorbtive, enteric factors synergizing insulin release, etc.). Figures 23, 24, and 25 depict mean levels of BG, IRI, and FFA seen in the same 11 controls and 5 prediabetics shown in Figures 17 and 18. As in the intravenous test, a high proportion of the individual tests showed statistically significant correlations between IRI and BG. An almost reciprocal change is seen comparing either BG or IRI to FFA levels.

Although no significant differences in mean BG or IRI levels were found comparing normals to prediabetics during either the intravenous or oral-loaded state, it was felt desirable to utilize the linear regression analysis data to evaluate the appropriateness of the IRI-BG relationship. Therefore, a pooled regression equation and slope constant was derived for the 11 controls during the intravenous and during the oral-loaded state, and a similar computation was derived for the 5 prediabetics. The plots of the linear regression equations during the oral test are shown in Figure 26. Smaller slope constants were seen in the prediabetics during both intravenous and oral testing, statistically significant for the oral test (p<0.01).

In summary, it can be stated that during two quite specific perturbations of "steady state" glucose homeostasis, a simple (and obviously incomplete) model has been made concerning IRI-BG relationships, and this model has been used to quantify the relationship. In the instances at hand, the quantification derived from the model has shown significant alterations in the relationship of the two parameters in an extremely early disease state prior to alterations in the absolute magnitude of either. The clinical conclusion that can be made on the basis of the analysis are consistent with findings shown by others in more severe degree of the disease (diabetes), and have been partially confirmed by a recent publication using a similar analysis of IRI-BG relationships [3, 20].

Furthermore, these analyses which indicate a blunted IRI response to glucose imply that this blunted IRI response might reflect normal or increased sensitivity of peripheral tissues to insulin as regards glucose uptake.

Further studies are in progress to quantify other types of glucose perturbations in the "overnight fasted, steady state" man. The quotation marks, as used here, are to indicate that the testing situation is really not truly fasted as described in the "Introduction" or in the "Steady State" using the true sense of the phrase. However, overnight fasted man does have what appears to be relatively constant magnitudes of BG and IRI over at least three to five-hour periods. As an example of such studies,

GLUCOSE HOMEOSTASIS

Figure 27 depicts levels of IRI and BG in a normal healthy subject prior to and during successive thirty-minute periods of constant glucose infusion at the rates shown. The following types of quantitative observations have been made [21].

A. Statistically significant elevations of serum IRI are seen when BG rises about 5 mgm% over the baseline level.

B. Statistically significant correlation exist between IRI and BG during both the slow ascending BG phase and the rapid descending phase of BG.

C. Estimations of the half-life of endogenous serum insulin computed during the descending IRI phase appear to be of the order of nine minutes.

D. The prediabetic subject shows a delay in the decline of serum IRI levels for five to ten minutes after the end of the glucose infusion [14].

These glucose infusion studies have extended the concept that IRI levels and possibly IRI secretion is directly related to BG levels [16]. However, other types or different formats of glucose administration have shown relatively greater IRI levels per BG level soon after initiation of the perturbation (two to ten minutes) when compared to later time intervals (twenty to sixty minutes) [10]. These data would therefore lend themselves to further modifications of the IRI-BG relationship analyses whereby a function of time could be included.

SUMMARY

In summary, a broad overview of fuel metabolism in man has been presented showing not only the interchange of fuel forms but also the differential regulatory effect of insulin upon various tissues. These essentially form a comprehensive set of "ground rules" for models of glucose homeostasis. In addition, a series of perturbations to the system have been shown for normal man and "prediabetic" man which have emphasized the clinical utility of hormone-fuel relationships. Finally, it would appear that the "glucose homeostasis" physiologist has now sufficient data in search of a mathematical model and that the biomathematician has a mathematical model in search of data. Melding of these two disciplines should be mutually symbiotic.

G.F. CAHILL, JR., AND J.S. SOELDNER

REFERENCES

1. Benedict, F.G. A Study of prolonged fasting. Carnegie Institute of Washington, publication 203, 1915.

2. Cahill, G.F., Jr., Herrera, M.G., Morgan, A.P., Soeldner, J.S., Steinke, J., Levy, P.L., Riechard, G.A., Jr. and Kipnis, D.M. Hormone-fule interrelationships during fasting. J.Clin. Invest. 45: 1751, 1966.

3. Colwell, J. and Lein, A. Diminished insulin response to hyperglycemia in pre-diabetes and diabetes. Diabetes 16: 560, 1967.

4. Crofford, O.B., Felts, P.W. and Lacy, W.W. Effect of glucose infusion on the individual plasma free amino acids in man. Proc. Soc. Exptl. Biol. Med. 117: 11, 1964.

5. Dupre, J. and Beck, J.C. Stimulation of release of insulin by an extract of intestinal mucosa. Diabetes 15: 555, 1966.

6. Exton, J.H. and Park, C.R. Control of gluconeogenesis in liver. I. General features of gluconeogenesis in the perfused liver of rats. J. Biol. Chem. 242: 2622, 1967

7. Floyd, J.C., Jr., Fajans, S.S., Conn, J.W., Knopf, R.F. and Rull, J. Insulin secretion in response to protein ingestion. J. Clin. Invest. 45: 1479, 1966.

8. Franckson, J.R.M. and Ooms, H. A., Bellens, R., Conard, V. and Bastenie, P.A. Physiologic significance of the intravenous glucose tolerance test. Metabolism 11: 482, 1962.

9. Goodman, A.D., Fuisz, R.E. and Cahill, G.F., Jr. Renal gluconeogenesis in acidosis, alkalosis, and potassium deficiency: Its possible role in the regulation of renal ammonia production. J. Clin. Invest. 45: 612, 1966.

10. Grodsky, G.M., Bennett, L.L., Smith, D.F. and Schmid, F.G. Effect of glucose or glucagon on insulin secretion in vitro. Metabolism 16: 222, 1967.

11. Herrera, M.G., Kamm, D., Ruderman, N. and Cahill, G.F., Jr. Non-hormonal factors in the control of gluconeogenesis in Advances in Advances in Enzyme Regulation, Weber, C., ed., 1966, Pergamon Press, Oxford and New York, p. 225.

12. Kamm, D.E., Fuisz, R.E., Goodman, A.D. and Cahill, G.F., Jr. Acid-base alterations and renal gluconeogenesis: Effect of pH, bicarbonate concentration, and pCO_2. J. Clin. Invest. 46: 1172, 1967.

13. Manchester, K.L. and Young, F.G. Hormones and protein biosynthesis in isolated rat diaphragm. J. Endocrinol. 18: 301, 1959.

14. Marble, A. Angiopathy in diabetes: an unsolved problem. Diabetes, to be published.

15. McIntyre, N., Holdsworth, C.D. and Turner, D.S. Intestinal factors in the control of insulin secretion. J. Clin. Endocr. 25: 1317, 1965.

16. Metz, R. The effect of blood glucose concentration on insulin output. Diabetes 9: 89, 1960.

17. Owen, O.E., Morgan, A.P., Kemp, H.G., Sullivan, J.M., Herrera, M.G. and Cahill, G.F., Jr. Brain metabolism during fasting. J. Clin. Invest. 46: 1589, 1967.

GLUCOSE HOMEOSTASIS

18. Rasio, E.A., Hampers, C.L., Soeldner, J.S. and Cahill, G.F., Jr. Diffusion of glucose, insulin, inulin, and Evans blue protein into thoracic duct lymph of man. J. Clin. Invest. 46: 903, 1967.

19. Samols, E., Marri, G. and Marks, V. Interrelationships of glucagon, insulin, and glucose. The insulinogenic effect of glucagon. Diabetes 15: 855, 1966.

20. Seltzer, H.S., Allen, E.W., Herron, A.L., Jr. and Brennon, M.T. Insulin secretion in response to glycemic stimulus. Relation of delayed initial release to carbohydrate intolerance in mild diabetes mellitus. J. Clin. Invest. 46: 323, 1967.

21. Williams, R.F., Gleason, R.E., Garcia, M.J. and Soeldner, J.S. Differences in the relationship between blood glucose and serum immunoreactive insulin during rapid and slow glucose infusions. Clin. Research 14: 356, 1966.

22. Williamson, J.R., Kreisberg, R.A. and Felts, P.W. Mechanism for the stimulation of gluconeogenesis by fatty acids in perfused rat liver. Proc. Nat. Acad. Sci. 56: 247, 1966.

23. Advances in Enzyme Regulation, Weber, G., ed., Volumes 1-6, 1963-1967, Pergamon Press, Oxford, and New York.

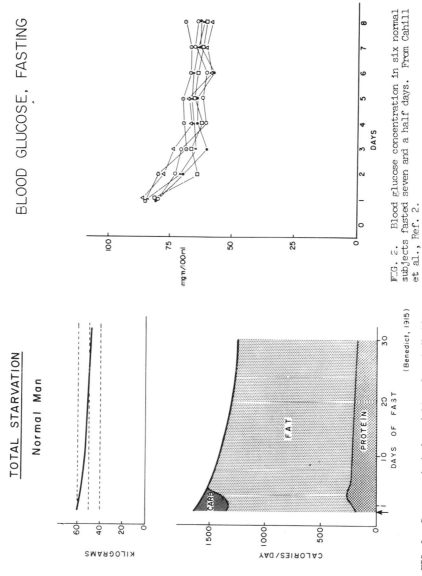

FIG. 2. Blood glucose concentration in six normal subjects fasted seven and a half days. From Cahill et al., Ref. 2.

FIG. 1. Decrease in body weight and contribution of carbohydrate, fat, and protein in a normal subject fasted for thirty days. Taken from Benedict, Ref. 1.

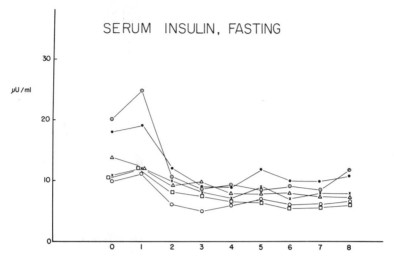

FIG. 3. Serum immunoreactive insulin in six normal subjects fasted seven and a half days. From Cahill et al., Ref. 2.

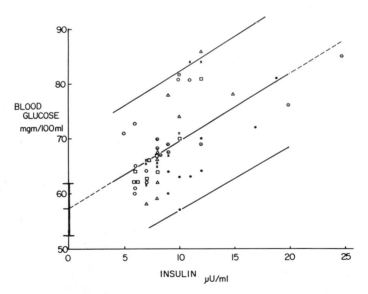

FIG. 4. Correlation of insulin and glucose levels taken from data in Figures 2 and 3. From Cahill et al., Ref. 2.

IV GTT BEFORE AND AFTER FAST

n = 6

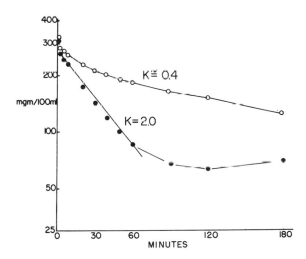

FIG. 5.   Glucose disappearance rate after
administration of glucose, 0.5 gram/kilogram, to
subjects after an overnight fast (solid circles)
and after seven and a half days of fasting
(open circles). Semilogarithmic plot with K
expressed as percent disappearing/minute. From
Cahill et al., Ref. 2.

SERUM IRI RESPONSE TO
IV GTT BEFORE AND
AFTER FAST

(n=6)

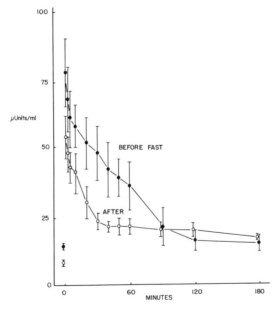

FIG. 6.   Mean serum immunoreactive responses ± standard
errors) in six normal subjects after an overnight fast
(labeled "before fast")and after seven and a half days
of total starvation (labeled "after").   From Cahill
et al., Ref. 2.

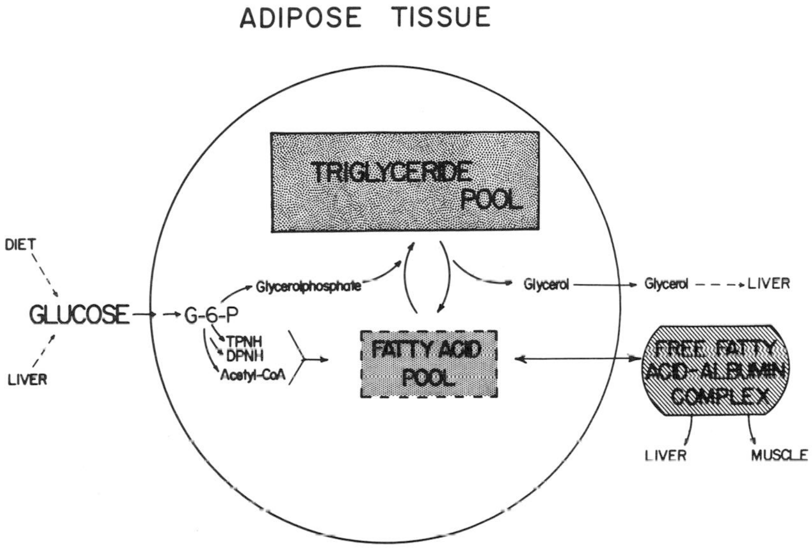

ADIPOSE TISSUE

FIG. 7. General scheme for metabolism in adipose tissue. Glucose
is metabolized to glucose-6-phosphate, which, in turn, is metabolized
to acetyl CoA and resynthesized into fatty acid and then esterified
with glycerolphosphate to form triglyceride. On hydrolysis of
triglyceride, free glycerol is produced and released. Free fatty
acids in the adipose tissue are in near equilibrium with the free
fatty acid albumin complex in the circulating fluids.

ADIPOSE TISSUE: INSULIN EFFECT

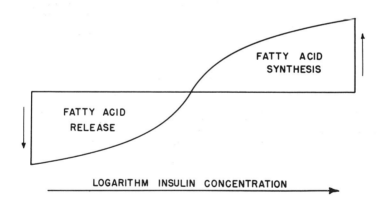

FIG. 8.   Schematic relationship of insulin and its effect in inhibiting free fatty acid release and promoting fatty acid synthesis.

G.F. CAHILL, JR., AND J.S. SOELDNER

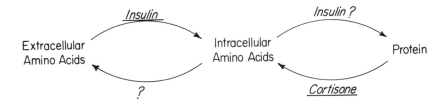

FIG. 9.   Relationship between extracellular and intracellular amino acids and tissue protein. Insulin promotes either amino acid transport or else directly protein synthesis. There is evidence for and against each step. In the absence of insulin, and in the presence of adrenal steroid, here labeled cortisone, there is a net proteolysis and release of amino acid.

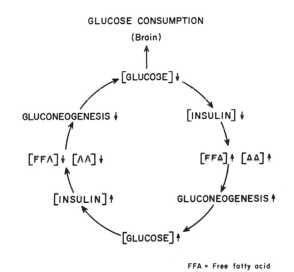

FIG 10.   Substrate-hormonal feedback relationships as described in the text.

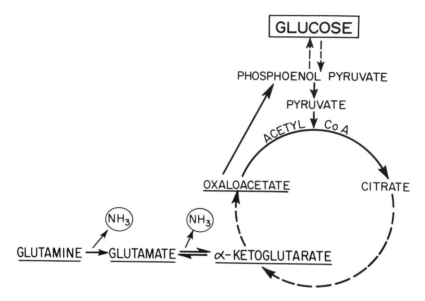

FIG. 11.   Relationship of ammonia production during acidotic states and rate of glucose production by kidney, a system apparently independent of direct hormonal control.

RELATIONSHIP OF BLOOD GLUCOSE TO LIVER GLUCOSE UPTAKE & PRODUCTION

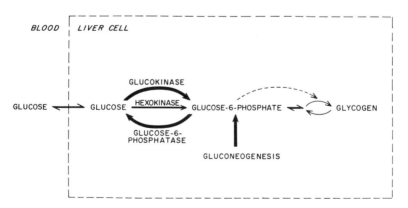

FIG. 12.   Enzymes involved in glucose, glucose-6-phosphate interrelations in liver.

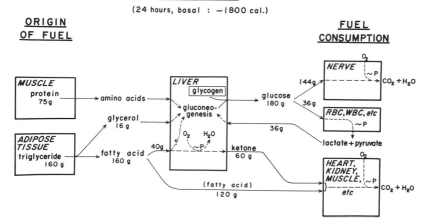

FIG. 13.   Overall scheme for fasting man – 24 hours.

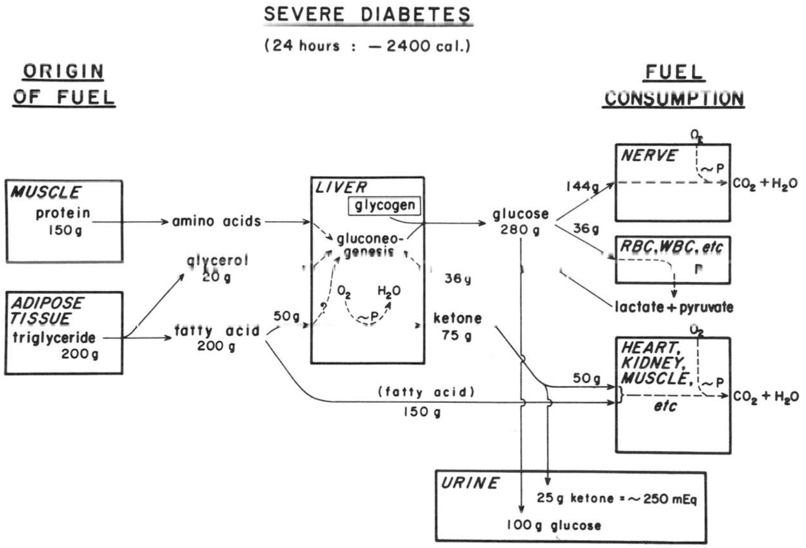

FIG. 14.   Overall scheme for "super-fasted" man – 24 hours – the situation in "insulin-lacking" or "severe diabetes."

GLUCOSE HOMEOSTASIS

FASTING MAN, ADAPTED (5-6 weeks)

(24 hours, basal : ~1500 calories)

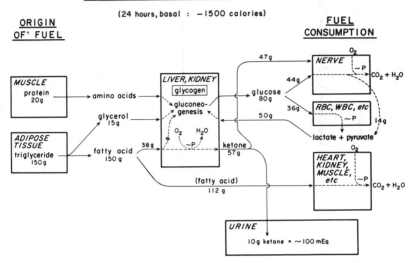

FIG. 15. Overall scheme for "fasted-adapted" man - 24 hours.

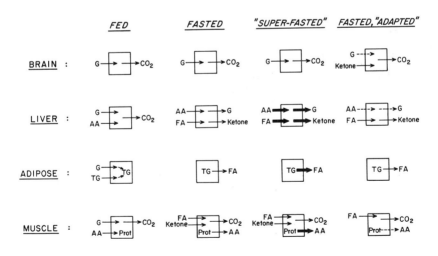

G = Glucose   AA = Amino Acid   FA = Fatty Acid   TG = Triglyceride   Prot = Protein

FIG. 16. Simplified scheme of substrate flow into and out of various organs in four metabolic states discussed in the text.

G.F. CAHILL, JR., AND J.S. SOELDNER

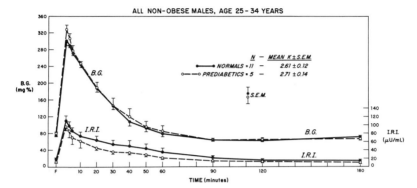

FIG. 17. Levels of blood glucose (B.G.) and serum immunoreactive insulin (I.R.I) during I.V. glucose tolerance tests (0.5 gm/kg)

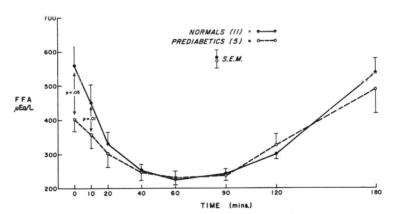

FIG. 18. Mean levels of plasma free fatty acids (FFA) during intravenous glucose tolerance tests (0.5 gm/kg Body Wt.)

GLUCOSE HOMEOSTASIS

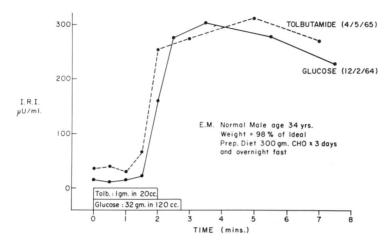

FIG. 19.   Levels of serum immunoreactive insulin (IRI) in contralateral
antecubital vein during and after rapid infusion of glucose (0.5 gm./kg.)
or tolbutamide (1 gm.)

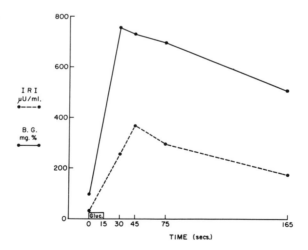

FIG. 20.   Mean levels of serum immunoreactive insulin (IRI)
and blood glucose (B.G.) in portal vein of 6 rats immediately
following glucose infusion (1.0 gm./kg.) in femoral vein

G.F. CAHILL, JR., AND J.S. SOELDNER

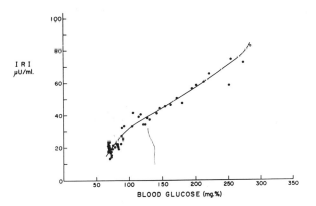

SAMPLES EVERY 2 MINS. FOR 120 MINS.

A.G. Normal Male age 30 yrs.
Weight = 112 % of Ideal
K = 2.33

FIG. 21.   Relationship of blood glucose and serum
immunoreactive insulin (IR) during rapid I.V. glucose
tolerance test (0.5 gm./kg.)

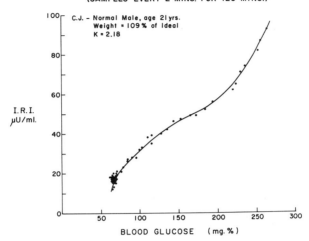

(SAMPLES EVERY 2 MINS. FOR 120 MINS.)

C.J. – Normal Male, age 21 yrs.
Weight = 109% of Ideal
K = 2.18

I.R.I.
μU/ml.

BLOOD GLUCOSE (mg. %)

FIG. 22. Relationship of blood glucose and serum immunoreactive insulin (IRI) during rapid I.V. glucose tolerance test (0.5 gm./kg.)

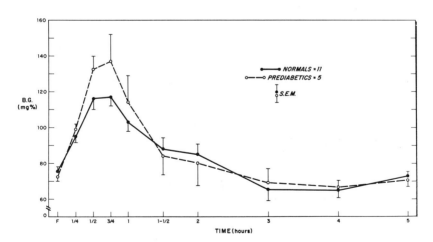

B.G.
(mg%)

NORMALS = 11
PREDIABETICS = 5
S.E.M.

TIME (hours)

FIG. 23. Mean levels of blood glucose during oral glucose tolerance test (100 gm). All non-obese males, age 25 – 34 years.

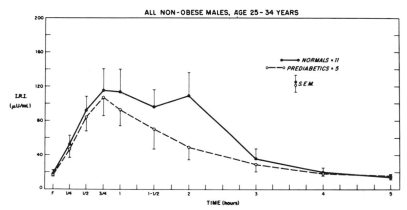

FIG. 24. Levels of serum immunoreactive insulin (I.R.I.) during oral glucose tolerance test (100 gm)

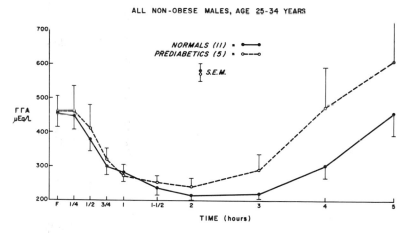

FIG. 25. Mean levels of plasma free fatty acids (FFA) during oral glucose tolerance tests (100 gm)

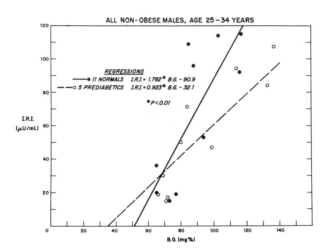

FIG. 26. Oral glucose tolerance test (100 gm). Mean levels of serum immunoreactive insulin (I.R.I.) at corresponding mean levels of blood glucose (B.G.)

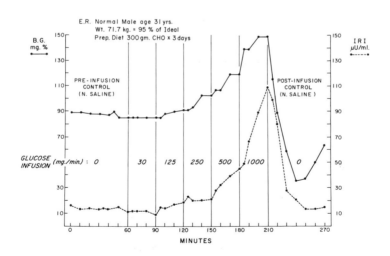

FIG. 27. Blood glucose (B.G.) and serum immunoreactive insulin (I.R.I.) response to glucose infusion (57 gm. in 2.5 hours)

4. MODELING AND CONTROL ASPECTS OF GLUCOSE HOMEOSTASIS

W.P. CHARETTE, A.H. KADISH and R. SRIDHAR
Department of Electrical Engineering, California Institute of Technology, Pasadena, California

MATHEMATICAL MODELS

Our remarks will begin with some general statements regarding mathematical modeling of physical and biological processes.

Mathematical modeling is associated with establishing reasonable mathematical representations which relate the stimuli (or inputs) to the responses (or outputs). Very often, stimuli and responses are defined subjectively. Moreover, the mathematical relationships depend to a great extent on the current state of development of mathematics as well as the areas of known mathematics with which the modeler is familiar and "comfortable".

The most common representation of hormonal control systems of the type under discussion here is in terms of differential or difference equations. This undoubtedly is greatly influenced by the use of differential equations in classical control theory.

The differential equation description of stimuli-response relations usually introduces intermediate variables called states. From a mathematical point of view the choice of states is not unique. However, this does not lead to any ambiguities in the stimuli-response relations. In biological applications it is often reasonable to make the states unique by insisting that they represent biologically meaningful entities. In some applications this is automatically taken care of when one uses a "multi-compartment" model, an approach which appears to be very popular in biological and physiological modeling.

It is evident that the very choice of differential equations for modeling implies subjective hypotheses. We shall focus further discussion on differential equation models even though many of the comments made here are equally pertinent

Supported in part by a grant from the John A. Hartford Foundation, New York, N.Y.

W.P. CHARETTE, A.H. KADISH AND R. SRIDHAR

for other types of mathematical representations.

The first matter for consideration is to decide whether a deterministic or stochastic model is appropriate for the phenomenon of interest. The appropriateness of a deterministic model is influenced by the "repeatability" of each of the experiments. Is it possible to conduct an experiment on the same subject under identical environmental conditions several times and observe identical responses? If this is not possible, then either a deterministic model is meaningless or all the causes which influence the model have not been taken into account.

Assuming that a model has been hypothesized, the next interesting question that arises is the so-called "inverse problem". This is the problem of determining the numerical values of the parameters in a model by suitably processing the data available on the stimuli and the associated response. This is a problem which is far from trivial even from the strictly theoretical point of view. The inverse problem is often complicated by questions of "observability". How can one be sure that the stimuli-response data contains enough information about the parameters? Or equivalently, how can one be sure that the response to the given stimulus is reasonably sensitive to changes in the values of the parameters?

Assuming that the inverse problem is meaningful and algorithms are available for its solution, the model should next satisfy certain predictability requirements. The model with parameters numerically determined based on the necessary response-stimuli data should yield predicted responses which can be corroborated experimentally for different types of stimuli.

Apparently the mathematical models proposed in the literature for glucose homeostasis focus mostly on the inverse problem, very little on repeatability, and not at all on predictability. Even the rather trivial predictions that can be made with linear models based on superposition seem to have been ignored.

METABOLIC CONTROL

Our current understanding of the interrelated processes and physical organs constituting the metabolic system and its endocrine control is depicted in the generic block diagram shown in Figure 1. This diagram represents an attempt on the part of the authors to systematize the following physiologic facts as a first step in the eventual derivation of a detailed metabolic control model using established engineering control systems concepts, theories, and techniques.

Under normal conditions the concentration of glucose in human plasma and extracellular fluid is maintained at approximately 100 mg/100 ml. This parameter is a product of interactions among (1) the state of the organism, (2) protein, lipid, and carbohydrate metabolism, and (3) the homeostatic control effected by hormones from the endocrine glands. These processes interact in such a fashion to closely regulate plasma glucose despite stresses upon the organism. The endocrine system controls the exchange between stored fuels, viz. protein, triglyceride, and glycogen, and their mobilized equivalents, viz. amino acids, triglyceride derivatives, and glucose respectively, so as to maintain the organism's homeostasis under varying environmental conditions.

The regulation of plasma glucose appears to be effected by two essentially distinct pathways. One is mediated through the pancreas which releases insulin when plasma glucose is above nominal and glucagon when plasma glucose is below nominal. The other is mediated through the hypothalamus and remaining endocrine glands, i.e. anterior hypophysis, adrenal, and thyroid, responding to a low or decreasing plasma glucose concentration. The nominal concentration is believed to be determined by the higher cortical centers of the central nervous system.

When the plasma glucose concentration rises to some point between 100 and 150 mg/100ml -- normally as a result of the ingestion of food -- the liver stops releasing glucose into plasma and begins to store the excess glucose as glycogen. Simultaneously the tissue utilization of glucose rises, adipose tissue stores glucose as triglyceride and muscle stores glucose as glycogen. When the concentration falls below nominal by approximately 5 to 10 mg/100 ml, growth hormone of the anterior hypophysis is released at an increased rate, promoting gluconcogenesis. The pancreas responds by releasing glucagon and the adrenal medulla by releasing epinephrine, both of which promote glycogenolysis and gluconeogenesis. Hydrocortisone from the adrenal cortex and triiodothyronine from the thyroid also are released under the stimulus of hypoglycemia. The evidence suggests that the pancreas and adrenal medulla perform comparator action directly, releasing their respective hormones as some function of glucose actuating error, whereas the hypothalamus plays this role for the remaining hormones. The hormone controller appears to respond as proportional, derivative, and integral functions of the actuating error between the nominal and actual plasma glucose concentration.

The overall system then includes a "plant" consisting of processes relating three metabolic fuel precursors (protein, triglyceride, glycogen) to three metabolic fuels (amino acids, triglyceride derivatives, glucose), three inputs (protein, fat, carbohydrate), one output (plasma glucose), and a "controller" producing six control signals (insulin, glucagon, epinephrine, growth hormone, hydrocortisone, triiodothyrone). To a control systems engineer it constitutes a nonlinear, multidimensional control system with normal and parametric feedback. The parametric feedback arises from the changes induced by hormones in specific enzyme-catalyzed reactions and membrane transport mechanisms thereby resulting in parametric changes

W.P. CHARETTE, A.H. KADISH AND R. SRIDHAR

to the dynamics associated with these processes and subsystems. In addition, many
of these processes exhibit saturation and threshold properties.

The translation of these statements into mathematics results in nonlinear differential equations. Hence the first step in systematizing the physiologic knowledge of
the metabolic system has led to the conclusion that the system is inherently nonlinear
and multidimensional. Any meaningful attempt to describe the system mathematically
cannot ignore these facts. The modeling problem is then to find mathematical representations for the detailed processes suggested by Figure 1 and to relate them in a
consistent manner resulting in an overall analytic representation of the metabolic
system. The above observations imply that a meaningful system model for metabolism
will involve nonlinear mathematics, hence the analytic diffculties implicit in these
efforts will necessitate the use of computation facilities for simulation purposes.
As will be seen in the sequel -- a literature survey of efforts to model the glucose
homeostatic system -- most of the reported work on this problem avoids the above mathematical difficulties by introducing assumptions which ignore either or both the multidimensional and nonlinear aspects of the problem.

CONTROL SYSTEMS AND GLUCOSE HOMEOSTASIS

Probably the first attempt to illustrate how the concepts of control systems engineering can be applied to the study of glucose homeostasis was supplied by Goldman
in 1960 [10]. In a qualitative fashion he summarized the major metabolic subsystems
and controlling hormones relevant to glucose regulation and represented their interconnection in a block diagram suggestive of a multi-loop feedback control system (see
Figure 2). Goldman did not attempt to develop his model in any more detail, but discussed the eventual application of modeling efforts in characterizing clinical abnormalities and in endocrine system research. Assuming that glucose regulation can
be viewed as a classical regulating system, Goldman emphasized the need for new experiments to understand the physiological mechanism of set-point establishment and
to identify which possible modes of control exist in this physiological system. Although Goldman's work does not enhance our physiological knowledge of glucose metabolism per se, it constitutes a logical first step in any detailed mathematical modeling of the system by identifying the major subsystems involved and their logical
interconnection in a systematic manner consistent with standard control system ter-
minology.

The next published work is that of Bolie [6,7] illustrating the use of analog
computers in simulation of mathematical representations of glucose regulation. The
first model treats the interaction of liever, kidney, pancreas, insulin, and glucose
in two compartments, the vascular and extravascular. The model is a gross simpli-

fication of the glucose regulating system, treating only one controlling hormone and being strictly linear except for a renal threshold. It qualitatively reproduces insulin and glucose behavior after simulated 6 minute infusions of glucose and insulin of 50 g. and 2 units respectively. The model is represented by Equations (1) through (4):

$$V_B \dot{I}_v = I_i + (I_e - I_v) P_I + K_1 G_v - K_2 I_v \qquad (1)$$

i.e., the rate of accumulation of insulin in the blood stream equals the rate of injection plus the rate of transfer from the extravascular compartment plus the rate at which it is released from the pancreas minus the rate at which it is degraded in the vascular compartment.

$$V_I \dot{I}_e = (I_v - I_e) P_I - K_3 I_e \qquad (2)$$

i.e., the rate of accumulation of insulin in the extravascular insulin space equals the rate of transfer from the vascular space minus the rate at which it is degraded in the extravascular space.

$$V_B \dot{G}_v = G_i + (G_e - G_v) P_G - f(G_v) - K_4 I_v - K_5 G_v \qquad (3)$$

i.e., the rate of accumulation of blood glucose equals the rate of injection plus the rate of transfer from the extravascular compartment minus renal excretion and storage in liver.

$$V_G \dot{G}_e = (G_v - G_e) P_G - K_6 I_e - K_7 G_e \qquad (4)$$

i.e., the rate of accumulation of extravascular glucose equals the rate of transfer from the vascular space minus tissue utilization.

Known nonlinear effects have been linearlized and represented by the constants K_1 through K_7. The renal nonlinearity $f(G_v)$ consists of a threshold and constant gain. Although the model does not yield any new information about glucose regulation, it does illustrate on a limited scale the use of simulation in verifying the consistency of a proposed model.

Bolie's second paper [7] neglects renal excretion and lumps the vascular system and extravascular system into one compartment. The model then reduces to two first-order linear differential equations:

W.P. CHARETTE, A.H. KADISH AND R. SRIDHAR

$$\dot{I} = \frac{I_1}{V} - \alpha I + \beta G \tag{5}$$

$$\dot{G} = \frac{G_1}{V} - \gamma I - \delta G \tag{6}$$

where (α) represents the sensitivity of insulinase activity to insulin concentration, (β) represents the sensitivity of pancreatic insulin output to glucose concentration, (γ) represents the combined sensitivity of liver glycogen storage and tissue glucose utilization to elevated insulin concentration, and (δ) represents the combined sensitivity of liver glycogen storage and tissue glucose utilization to elevated glucose concentration.

The parameters of this model were derived from data obtained from various sources, in some cases values were "averaged" across species! No attempt was made to verify the behavior of the model by predictability of experiments. It is evident that at best the model parameters are chosen optimally with respect to one experiment.

The next published effort in modeling of glucose regulation is that of Seed, Acton, and Stunkard. [13] The model relates liver, kidney, brain, pancreas, vascular and extravascular compartments, and a substance Z, presumably related to insulin, in terms of three dependent variables connected by piecewise linear ordinary differential equations. The equations represent respectively, the rate of change of glucose in the "fast" compartment, the rate of change of glucose in the "slow" compartment, and the rate of change of substance Z in the liver. The expressions in square brackets are zero unless the condition note below each bracket is satisfied.

$$\dot{G}_f = -D_f G_f + D_s G_s - L_z G_f - M_a G_f - B - [M_f G_f - m_f] - [R G_f - r] + [p_g - P_g Z] + [I]$$

$$\{G_f > L_f\} \qquad \{G_f > L_v\} \qquad \{Z < L_p\} \qquad \{t < L_T\} \tag{7}$$

$$\dot{G}_s = D_f G_f - D_s G_s - [M_s G_s - m_s] \tag{8}$$

$$\{G_s > L_s\}$$

$$\dot{Z} = -c_z - C_z Z + F_z G_f \tag{9}$$

These equations were simulated and by trial and error parameter adjustment showed qualitative agreement over a limited interval with some kind of an "average" of plasma glucose after a 25 g. infusion taken over 70 normal subjects (see Figure 3). These data were obtained by Amatuzio. [3] However, this method of model verification was found to yield physiologically unrealistic parameters.

These investigators then expanded the model to include two new compartments, red blood cells and plasma. The equations represent, respectively, the rate of change of plasma glucose, fast compartment glucose, slow compartment glucose, red blood cell glucose, and substance Z in liver.

$$\dot{G}_p = - (D_{pf}G_p - D_{fp}G_f) - (D_{ps}G_p - D_{sp}G_s) - KV_{G_c} \quad \frac{G_p}{G_p + G_{\phi_p}} - \frac{G_c}{G_c + G_{\phi_c}}$$

$$-[\Gamma_g Z - p_g] - L_z G_f - [RG_p - r] - B + [I] \tag{10}$$

$$\{Z < L_p\} \qquad \{G_p > L_r\} \; \{t < L_T\}$$

$$\dot{G}_f - (D_{pf}G_p - D_{fp}G_f) - M_a G_f - [M_f G_f - m_f] \tag{11}$$

$$\{G_f > L_f\}$$

$$\dot{G}_s = (D_{ps}G_p - D_{sp}G_s) - M_b G_s - [M_s G_s - m_s] \tag{12}$$

$$\{G_s > L_s\}$$

$$\dot{G}_c = KV_{G_c} \quad \frac{G_p}{G_p + G_{\phi_p}} - \frac{G_c}{G_c + G_{\phi_c}} \tag{13}$$

$$\dot{Z} = F_z G_f - [C_z Z + c_z]$$

$$\{Z > 0\}$$

W.P. CHARETTE, A.H. KADISH AND R. SRIDHAR

The authors attempted to substantiate all parameter values from published experimental results before computer simulations were undertaken. Again, roughly qualitative reproduction of experimental results was obtained, and it was concluded that
more knowledge of glucose metabolism was required before a more refined model could
be postulated. In view of the more recent results obtained in hormone effects and
the fact that these are not included in this work, the deficiencies of the model are
substantial. As in the previous two efforts, the model amounts to a more sophisticated attempt at curve-fitting.

In 1962 Beliles [4] evaluated by experiments on dogs the coefficients in the
Bolie model (Equations (5) and (6)). In addition he proposed a five-compartment model consisting of first-order linear ordinary differential equations and discussed
preliminary estimates of the parameters. The compartments consist of arterial blood,
pancreas, liver, splanchnic area minus pancreas and liver, and peripheral tissue.

A schematic illustrating the model is shown in Figure 4. The detailed equations
of the model are given by (16) through (34), but they can be represented by the vector equation:

$$\dot{x} = Ax + f \tag{15}$$

where x is eight-dimensional .

Insulin and glucose concentrations in the extracellular fluid of peripheral tissue are represented by:

$$\dot{I}_b = - \frac{F_b}{V_b} [I_b - I_a] \tag{16}$$

$$\dot{G}_b = - \frac{F_b}{V_b} [G_b - G_a] - \frac{M_b}{V_b} \tag{17}$$

The concentrations of insulin and glucose in pancreas efferent blood are represented
by:

$$\dot{I}_p = - \frac{F_p}{V_p} [I_p - I_a] + \frac{R}{V_p} \tag{18}$$

$$\dot{G}_p = - \frac{F_p}{V_p} [G_p - G_a] - \frac{M_p}{V_p} \tag{19}$$

The concentrations of insulin and glucose in splanchnic tissues efferent blood are represented by:

$$\dot{I}_s = -\frac{F_s}{V_s}\,[I_s - I_a] \tag{20}$$

$$\dot{G}_s = -\frac{F_s}{V_s}\,[G_s - G_a] - \frac{M_s}{F_s} \tag{21}$$

And the concentrations of insulin and glucose in the liver efferent blood are represented by:

$$\dot{I}_\ell = -\frac{F}{V_\ell}\,[-\,I_\ell + I_\omega] - \frac{D}{V_\ell} \tag{22}$$

$$\dot{G}_\ell = -\frac{F_\ell}{V_\ell}\,[-\,G_\ell + G_\omega] - \frac{H}{V_\ell} \tag{23}$$

It can be seen that blood flow rates are related by:

$$F_p + F_s = F_\ell \tag{24}$$

$$F_\ell + F_b = F_t$$

Continuity of transport rates requires that:

$$F_p I_p + F_s I_s = F_\ell I_\omega \tag{25}$$

$$F_p G_p + F_s G_s = F_\ell G_\omega \tag{26}$$

$$F_\ell G_\ell + F_b G_b = F_t G_a \tag{27}$$

$$F_\ell I_\ell + F_b I_b = F_t I_a \tag{28}$$

Insulin production is linearly related to circulating glucose:

$$R = K_r G_p \tag{29}$$

W.P. CHARETTE, A.H. KADISH AND R. SRIDHAR

Destruction of insulin by the liver is made proportional to the concentration of insulin leaving the liver:

$$D = K_b I_\ell \tag{30}$$

Storage of glucose by the liver is made linearly proportional to glucose and insulin levels above some minimal levels:

$$H = H_o + K_{\ell_1}(G_1 + G_o) + K_{\ell_2}(I_1 - I_o) \tag{31}$$

The rates of metabolism of glucose in peripheral tissue, splanchnic area and pancreas are represented by:

$$M_b = M_{b_o} + K_{b_1}(G_b - G_1) + K_{b_2}(I_b - I_1) \tag{32}$$

$$M_s = M_{s_o} + K_{s_1}(G_s - G_2) + K_{s_2}(I_s - I_2) \tag{33}$$

$$M_p = M_{p_o} + K_{p_1}(G_p - G_3) + K_{p_2}(I_p - I_3) \tag{34}$$

Parameter values were obtained from published experimental results. No attempt was made to compare the performance of this linear time-invariant model with actual experimental data. Because of the linear form of the equations and some of the simplifying assumptions made, e.g., inclusion of only insulin as a controlling hormone, at best the model could have only limited success in representing the regulation of glucose.

As we have seen, Bolie's work resulted in a model which can be represented by the vector equation:

$$\dot{x} = Ax + f + g \tag{35}$$

where x, f and g are 4-vectors and A is a 4 x 4 constant matrix. The 4 components of x represent glucose and insulin concentrations in plasma and outside plasma, f includes a nonlinearity for renal excretion and g represents glucose and insulin infusions. Bolie then reduced the order of the system by two to emphasize intravascular glucose and insulin coefficients, i.e.,

$$\dot{x} = Ax + g \tag{36}$$

where x and g are 2-vectors and A is a 2 x 2 constant matrix. The g vector again represents glucose and insulin infusion.

In 1963 Wrede [16] extended these results to a linear model representing glucose metabolism as a function of the hormones insulin, glucagon, epinephrine, cortisol, thyroxin and growth hormone. His model can be represented:

$$\dot{x} = Ax + f \tag{37}$$

where x is a 7-vector representing plasma concentration of glucose and the six hormones under consideration; A is a 7 x 7 constant matrix; and f is a 7-vector representing infusion rates of glucose and six hormones.

Wrede attempted to derive the parameters of the model, i.e., the coefficients of the A matrix in (37), from the available experimental data. The author recognized that a desired goal in modeling is a physiologically meaningful representation in contrast to "curve-fitting". Because of the linearity of the model, all of the substantial body of control systems analysis techniques could be brought to bear on the problem. By striving for equation consistency and analyzing how equilibrium constraints dictate model behavior, he was able to establish theoretical values for the parameters that could not be obtained from the available experimental data.

Analysis of the model yielded numerical values for certain parameters which are remarkably close to the experimentally determined values, tending to lend credence to the results. However, of more interest is the fact that this model for the first time predicted physiological consequences that had not been experimentally corroborated at that time. It is, of course, also possible that these conclusions are anomalous artifacts resulting from inadequacies of the model. However, this work does demonstrate how model building and simulation can enhance research in these physiological processes. Finally, the author simulated glucose and insulin tolerance tests on the model which yielded qualitatively reasonable behavior for some of the components of x.

Although the limitations in Wrede's model are clearly evident, his is the first attempt at constructing a model that includes all of the known hormonal controls believed to affect glucose metabolism. All such efforts prior to Wrede considered only the effects of insulin, whereas he considered the effects of six hormones, albeit in a linear fashion only.

In 1964 McLean [12] published a brief summary of glucose homeostasis focusing primarily on Goldman's [10] work. He attempted to incorporate nervous system effects explicitly in a modified system block diagram. However, owing to our very rudimentary understanding of mathematical representations for neural processes,

W.P. CHARETTE, A.H. KADISH AND R. SRIDHAR

successful modeling of such processes await the results of more basic research.

Keeping in mind the complexity of the overall metabolic control system as depicted in Figure 1 we see that the above reported results are representative attempts at achieving some kind of a mathematical representation for certain portions of the complete system. Common to these efforts.is a restricted emphasis on glucose metabolism, lipid and protein metabolism being neglected.

Although not representative of metabolic system modeling, some related work has been done on glucose tolerance test analysis by Ackerman and coworkers [1,2]. They sought to characterize a subject's response to a glucose input by one parameter in an attempt to identify normal or abnormal system behavior on the basis of the parameter value. Basically, their approach uses a linear second order model and the natural frequency of oscillation of the model is the parameter under study. The system variables are glucose and insulin concentration in blood. For the categorization of a specific subject, a glucose tolerance test is performed and the ensuing blood glucose concentration is sampled at a finite set of points over an interval of 180 min. The parameters of the model are fitted to this data in a least-squares sense. The resultant parameters then dictate a value for ω_o, the natural frequency of the glucose regulation model (presumably also that of the subject). On the basis of experiments on many subjects they concluded that classification of normals vs. diabetics in terms of ω_o was comparable in reliability to previously used techniques. However, they also recognize that borderline cases are difficult to classify. [2]

An analytically motivated diagnostic technique will hopefully eventually result from successful efforts at metabolic control system modeling. Considering the complexity of the system however, it would be rather surprising if a useful tool could result from the least-squares fit of a second order equation to the coarsely sampled response of the metabolic system to a glucose input.

In 1965 Shames [14] reported on a mathematical model for the dynamic response of glucose in extracellular fluid and intracellular hepatic fluid, insulin in plasma and interstitial fluid, and FFA in extracellular fluid to a glucose input (Equations (38) to (42)).

$$V_e \dot{G}_e = s_1 + k_1(G_\ell - G_e) - k_2(G_e - G_{tm}) - B - [k_3 + k_4 I_i + k_5(F_b - F_e)](G_e - G_t) \tag{38}$$

$$V_\ell \dot{G}_\ell = b_1 - k_6 I_p \ \overline{G_\ell + M_{p\ell}} \ -k_1(G_\ell - G_e) \tag{39}$$

$$V_p \dot{I}_p = b_2 + k_7 G_e^2 - k_8(I_p - I_i) - k_9 I_p \tag{40}$$

$$V_1 \dot{I}_1 = k_8(I_p - I_1) - k_{10}I_1 \tag{41}$$

$$V_e \dot{F}_e = b_3 - k_{11} \{[k_3 + k_4 I_1 + k_5(F_b - F_e)](G_e - G_t) - P_b\} - k_{12}F_e \tag{42}$$

Pancreatic insulin production is made proportional to the square of extracellular glucose and exchange between the plasma and the interstitial space is by simple diffusion (see Equations (40) and (41)). Equation (39) reflects the fact that simple diffusion relates extracellular fluid glucose and hepatic intracellular fluid glucose and the assumption that the Michaelis-Menten kinetics of the hexokinose-glucose-6-phosphatase system are rapidly changed to produce net phosphorylation by plasma insulin through a constant. Both removal of FFA through oxidation and recycling through adipose tissue stores are represented by a linear process and lumped into the constant k_{12}. The rate of decrease of FFA is proportional through k_{11} to the increase in the rate of peripheral utilization of glucose above the basal rate. These effects are represented by Equation (42). Equation (38), representing sources and sinks for glucose, contains the hepatic term as in Equation (39), a sink linearly related to glucose concentration above a threshold for renal excretion, a constant for CNS utilization, and a term linearly related to the extracellular fluid-peripheral tissue intracellular fluid gradient weighted by insulin and FFA concentrations.

It was the intent of the author to study some aspects of glucose regulation from a theoretical systems viewpoint using experimental data in the reported literature. Although the model treats only one aspect of the glucose regulatory system, that pertaining to an elevated glucose condition, the author fully appreciates the limitations of his methods, eg. combining into the model data from both in vitro and in vivo experiments in animals and man, and understands the role of systems techniques in such investigations. This is the first reported attempt to include in a model of glucose control the effects of FFA. It constitutes a correct step forward toward the mathematical representation of the full metabolic control system depicted in Figure 1, of which the glucose control system per se forms only a part.

Early in 1967 Cerasi published the results of some work done in Sweden on analog simulation of glucose regulation. [8] The model represents insulin and glucose in one compartment and includes renal excretion, peripheral glucose uptake, and insulin secretion. The release of insulin in response to glucose concentration is represented in two phases, the release of stored insulin and the release of newly formed insulin. The model is not strictly linear, since the uptake rate of glucose by peripheral tissue, for example, is represented as proportional to the product of

W.P. CHARETTE, A.H. KADISH AND R. SRIDHAR

insulin and glucose concentrations, and a renal excretion threshold is included.
The author claims successful simulation of many experimental tests performed on humans in the hospital laboratories. However, it is apparent that the model is an
insufficient representation of the glucose regulatory system, considering what is
known today about the metabolic processes involved and the attendant humoral controls. The basic purpose of the author was to represent in a mathematical fashion
the behavior of glucose and insulin concentration after a glucose load by means of
a lumped model.

Some more recent work on glucose modeling is due to Wolaver. [15] His model is
in terms of our first-order nonlinear differential equations depicting the behavior
of glucose and insulin in two compartments, the vascular and the extravascular, i.e.

$$V_B \frac{d}{dt} (BG) = f_L(BG,BI) - f_R(BG) + P_G(CG-BG) \tag{43}$$

$$V_G \frac{d}{dt} (CG) = P_G(BG-CG) - f_U(BG,BI) \tag{44}$$

$$V_B \frac{d}{dt} (BI) = f_P(BG) - (K)(BI) + P_I(CI-BI) \tag{45}$$

$$V_I \frac{d}{dt} (CI) = P_I(BI-CI) - (KD)(CI) \tag{46}$$

Wolaver attempts to obtain reasonable numbers for as many parameters as possible
from published experimental data, and determines the remainder by fitting the model
response to experimental results. The author recognizes some weaknesses of the model such as the questionable practice of extrapolating animal data to humans and
the gross lumping of hormonal effects into one control signal called "insulin". In
addition he discusses the use of models in establishing auxiliary control for diabetics through the use of a model reference adaptive system and the application of
optimal control theory for synthesizing such auxiliary control mechanisms.

The authors of this review have been working on a mathematical description of
the system in humans that maintains a prescribed concentration of glucose in circulation. The ultimate objective is for a detailed model of the system functionally
represented in Figure 1 which includes the coupling relationships among proteins,
lipids, and carbohydrates in metabolism.

A somewhat different approach in this work has been followed by the authors in contrast to that surveyed above. Owing to the complexity of the system depicted in Figure 1 and the paucity of experimental data that can suggest reasonably valid analytical models for the relevant subsystems, we have tried to construct models using as small a set of basic analytical building blocks as possible with parameter values chosen for any specific process within a given class to accommodate the behavior of that process. The real objective in this work is to demonstrate by means of examples what control systems techniques can contribute to our understanding of these biological regulation systems. Although a great amount of physiology has yet to be learned about the relevant subsystems involved before a definitive model can be established, it is our belief that the systems analyst can contribute to this effort now by systematizing our knowledge about the metabolic system in a consistent mathematical framework, by suggesting to the physiologist specific experiments suggested by model building, simulation, and analysis, and by determining analytically the dynamical consequences of conflicting theories concerning the operation of specific portions of the system.

Beginning with the recognition that the system contains inherent nonlinearities such as saturation effects and threshold phenomena, the models are constructed from first order nonlinear differential equations. All the models are simulated by digital computer and compared to actual data on humans in controlled experiments.

In August 1967 the authors presented a report on some preliminary results in modeling of hormonal control of glucose metabolism. [9] This work treated the glucose loop with two controlling hormones, insulin and glucagon (see Figure 5). The system is considered to be that of a normal, 70 kg unstressed adult subject; sex hormones are neglected. Initial conditions are intended to depict a normal human plasma glucose regulator in steady-state, i.e., in metabolic and endocrine equilibrium, hence parameter dependencies are represented in terms of deviations from the nominal.

Hormone generation is modeled on the basis of the sequence, secretion, accumulation, and depletion. Physiologically, hormone secretion rates monotonically increase from nominal until saturation occurs. This action is modeled by the smooth and symmetric nonlinearity:

$$r = r_o + \alpha \tanh [\beta(e-e_o)] \qquad (47)$$

where r is the hormone secretion rate in [mas/unit time] and e is the stimulus. This particular analytic form was chosen with a view to simplifying the inverse or identification problem, which amounts to either a parameter optimization or two-point boundary value problem if α and β are assumed constant. The function (47)

W.P. CHARETTE, A.H. KADISH AND R. SRIDHAR

reproduces the so-called "hyperbolic" behavior of first-order Michaelis-Menten rate kinetics and the so-called "sigmoid" behavior of a series of such reactions with sufficient accuracy until more precise analytic forms are justified by physiological data. Such functions are used to model glycogenolysis, glycogenesis, insulin secretion and glucagon secretion. Following several investigators, the effect of hormones on the function (47) is modeled as a linear change to the saturation value of the nonlinearity. For example:

$$r = r_o + \alpha \tanh [\beta(e-e_o)] \tag{48}$$

$$r_o = (r_h + r_\ell)/2$$

$$\alpha_o = (r_h - r_\ell)/2 \tag{49}$$

$$r_h = \gamma h + r_{ho} \tag{50}$$

where h is the pertinent hormone concentration affecting the lumped rate kinetics (47), and γ is a constant. Accumulation and depletion are modeled by first-order kinetics, in which it is assumed that the degradation rate is proportional to the concentration, i.e.

$$\dot{h} = -k_2 h + k_1 r \tag{51}$$

where k_2 has dimension [1/unit time] and k_1 has dimension [1/unit volume]. The parameters k_1 and k_2 have been measured by various techniques, eg. radioactive tracers, for several hormones, k_1 representing the circulatory volume and k_2 the degradation factor.

Consider the problem of establishing parameter values for the following hormone model based on physiological data.

$$\dot{h} = -k_2 h + k_1 [r + f_e] \tag{52}$$

$$r = r_o + \alpha \tanh[\beta(e-e_o)]$$

where f_e represents an exogenous input of the hormone h. Suppose the hormone under consideration is insulin, where (47) represents the generation and release of insulin from the pancreas into the plasma. Then we must identify k_1, k_2, r_o, α, β, and e_o. Theoretically the identification can be carried out in two steps. We will assume perfect observations to simplify the illustration.

If we administer $f_e(t)$, a known quantity of insulin intravenously, the resulting hypoglycemic state implies that $r = 0$ in (52), i.e. the endogenous production of insulin is at or below its nominal value. Adjoining the parameters k_1 and k_2 to the differential equation (52) we obtain,

$$\dot{h} = -k_2 h + k_1 f_e$$

$$\dot{k}_1 = 0 \tag{53}$$

$$\dot{k}_2 = 0$$

Given the input $f_e(t)$, $0 \leq t \leq T$ and three measurements of $h(t)$, $h(t_i)$, $i = 1,2,3$, these data and (53) constitute a multipoint boundary value problem which can be solved for k_1 and k_2 by the technique of quasilinearization, for example. [5] After each iteration the specific k_1 and k_2 obtained are substituted into (52) and the equation integrated to yield $\bar{h}(t)$, $0 \leq t \leq T$. Given some $c > 0$, the process is repeated until some criterion such as,

$$\sum_{i=1}^{3} [h(t_i) - \bar{h}(t_i)]^2 < \varepsilon \tag{54}$$

is satisfied.

Now assuming k_1 and k_2 fixed, and $f_e(t) \equiv 0$, a glucose input can be administered dictating $c(t)$, $0 \leq t \leq T$. Identifying r_o, e_o, α, and β can now theoretically be done in a similar manner with a minimum of six measurements on $h(t)$ by solving,

W.P. CHARETTE, A.H. KADISH AND R. SRIDHAR

$$\dot{h} = -k_2 h + k_1 \{r_o + \alpha \tanh[\beta(e-e_o)]\}$$

$$\dot{r} = \alpha \beta \operatorname{sech}^2[\beta(e-e_o)] \dot{e}$$

$$\dot{\alpha} = 0 \tag{55}$$

$$\dot{\beta} = 0$$

$$\dot{r}_o = 0$$

$$\dot{e}_o = 0$$

and satisfying and expression such as (54).

Returning to the discussion of the first glucose regulation model derived by the authors (Figure 5), it can be more compactly written as follows:

$$\dot{c} = -K_{19}c + K_{18}[F + f_{LO}(c,x_2) - f_{LU}(c,x_1,y_3) - f_R(c) - f_U(c,x_1) - GU] \tag{56}$$

$$\dot{x}_1 = -K_8 x_1 + K_7[I + f_1(c)] \tag{57}$$

$$\dot{x}_2 = -K_{11}x_2 + K_{10}[G + f_2(c)] \tag{58}$$

where:

$$c = \text{plasma glucose concentration}$$

$$x_1 = \text{plasma insulin concentration}$$

$$x_2 = \text{plasma glucagon concentration}$$

$$y_3 = \text{liver glycogen content}$$

$$F = \text{intravenous glucose input rate}$$

$$GU = \text{central nervous system mean glucose utilization rate}$$

$$I = \text{intravenous insulin input rate}$$

$$G = \text{intravenous glucagon input rate}$$

$$f_{LO}(c,x_2) = \text{liver glucose output rate}$$

$$f_{LU}(c,x_1,y_3) = \text{liver glucose uptake rate}$$

$$f_R(c) = \text{renal excretion rate}$$

$f_U(c,x_1)$ = peripheral tissue glucose utilization rate dependent on insulin

K_{19} = hormone independent tissue utilization rate coefficient

Numerical values for the model parameters were first obtained by reasoning from
results in the biologic, physiologic, and medical literature. Refinements were made
by simulating experiments in which glucose or insulin were administered under controlled conditions. An intravenous injection of glucose or insulin appears to the
system as an impulse function. It was found that a finite duration step function
was an adequate representation of such a test input. Simulations which corresponded
to tests ranging in duration from one to six hours in real time were performed.

An experiment [11] was performed on a normal adult subject in which ten units
of insulin were administered at the start, plasma glucose was continuously monitored,
and depending upon the monitored plasma glucose concentration varying quantities of
glucose were injected every two minutes in an attempt to manually maintain the subject's plasma glucose at or near nominal for a period of 100 minutes. The monitor
has an inherent time delay of approximately eight minutes. The system glucose response is shown in Figure 6 and the administered glucose input is shown in Figure 7.
The effect of the equipment time delay in such a control scheme is clearly evident
in Figure 6. The initial rise in the response is due to trace amounts of glucagon
in the initial intravenous injection of insulin.

This experiment was simulated with the model of Figure 5. Before this particular simulation was undertaken the parameters of the model were chosen to reproduce
experimental results due to a glucose input alone and an insulin input alone. These
parameters were then viewed as more or less constrained and a simulation of the data
in Figure 6 was sought such that the model's simulation of a glucose or insulin input was not deteriorated from that obtained previously. The simulation results are
shown in Figure 8. Other choices of parameters yielded a closer match to the actual
response, but resulted in less than satisfactory glucose alone or insulin alone responses. The response shown was obtained with circulation volumes for glucose, insulin, and glucagon of 26, 7, and 14 liters respectively (k_{18}, k_7, and k_{10}), degradation factors of .07, .03, and .222 respectively (k_{19}, k_8, and k_{11}) corresponding to time constants of 14.43, 33.33, and 4.5 minutes respectively. Physiologic
considerations dictate circulation volumes within a factor of about two and the same
can be said of degradation factors based on tracer experiments. The maximum freedom
in choice of parameters was found to lie in the area of greatest physiologic variation, via. parameter values for the nonlinearities $f_{LU}(c,x_1,y_3)$ the rate of uptake
of glucose by liver as a function of glucose error and insulin concentration, and

W.P. CHARETTE, A.H. KADISH AND R. SRIDHAR

$f_U(c,x_1)$ the rate of glucose utilization by tissue under the influence of insulin.

The rather large difference between data and simulation in the period $0 \le t < 30$ minutes (see Figure 8) was corrected by incorporating a first order lag with a time constant of 15. minutes to account for circulation dynamics.

Although this crude model does not adequately reproduce the finer details of the actual response this limited success supports the general approach to the problem and a belief that the inclusion of the remaining hormonal controls as well as more complex control laws will yield better results.

As an illustration of how control systems techniques can improve experimental methods, the above experiment, in which the human experimenter inserts himself in the control loop to administer glucose after observing the subjects's response to an insulin input, was simulated with the model described above and a simple control law of the following type was used to determine the control function, $F(t)$.

$$F(t) = K_1 \, c(t) + K_2 \, \frac{dc(t)}{dt} + K_3 \int_o^t c(t) \, dt \qquad (59)$$

No attempt was made to optimize some criterion function of glucose deviation from nominal, but the coefficients in (59) were selected by simulation to obtain better control than that which was achieved manually. With $K_1 = -200$, $K_2 = -50$, and $K_3 = -10$, the simulated response in Figure 9 was obtained. The required F(t) yielding this system response is illustrated in Figure 10 and the simulated insulin response is illustrated in Figure 11. If the model used in this simulation is representative of the dynamics of the real system - Subject Z - then we would expect that the experiment - 10^u regular insulin administered at $t = 0$ - repeated with the glucose input policy illustrated in Figure 10 will yield better results than those obtained when the glucose input policy (see Figure 7) was manually determined, i.e. the experiment should now yield a response more similar to the dotted line in Figure 9.

The model more recently under consideration still focuses on glucose metabolism, but with four controlling hormones, insulin, glucagon, epinephrine, and growth hormone. The model for the metabolic plant is shown in Figure 12, depicting the control of liver function, renal function, muscle and adipose tissue utilization of glucose, by four controlling hormones through parametric feedback, in a one-compartment configuration. The model being used for the four-component hormonal controller is shown in Figure 13 and includes both proportional and rate sensitive control modes.

The signals for hormone action are taken to be glucose error and error rate.

The model can also be represented as follows:

$$\tau_{18}\ddot{c}_1 + \dot{c}_1 = G_{18}[F(t-\tau_1) + f_{LO}(c_1,h_2,h_3) - f_{LU}(c_1,x_4,h_1) - f_R(c_1) - G_9 c_1 -$$

$$f_M(x_{11}) - f_L(x_{11},h_4)] \tag{60}$$

$$\dot{h}_1 = - K_6 h_1 + K_5 \{K_1(h_3)[f_1(c_1) + f_2(\dot{c}_1)] + I(t-\tau_2)\} \tag{61}$$

$$\dot{h}_2 = - K_{11}h_2 + K_{10}[f_3(c_1) + G(t-\tau_3)] \tag{62}$$

$$\dot{h}_3 = - K_{21}h_3 + K_{20}[f_4(c_1) + f_5(\dot{c}_1) + E(t-\tau_4)] \tag{63}$$

$$\dot{h}_4 = - K_{31}h_4 + K_{30}[f_6(c_1) + S(t-\tau_5)] \tag{64}$$

$$\text{where:} \quad x_{11}(t) = \frac{G_7}{\tau_7} \int_0^t e^{-(t-\tau)/\tau_7} h_1(\tau)d\tau \tag{65}$$

The parameters of this model were adjusted to simulate the results of two experiments. In the first, 15 g. of glucose was infused over 3 minutes in a normal male subject, and in the second, 5^u of regular insulin was injected at $t = 0$ followed by 1 mg of glucagon at $t = 58$ minutes; the results of the simulations are shown in Figures 14 and 15 respectively.

Using the same parameter values resulting from the above in the model, a 30 g. infusion of glucose over three minutes was simulated. The comparison of the model predicted behavior with the subject's response to this new input is depicted in Figure 16.

The above modeling effort is being extended to encompass the two other major metabolic subsystems of Figure 1, lipid metabolism and protein metabolism. At the same time, mathematical approaches to solving the inverse problem are being investigated.

Results of model comparison with experiments enforce the belief that only high dimension nonlinear models will yield a sufficiently accurate description of the operation of complex metabolic processes and their endocrine control. We recognize that even though our efforts at modeling these processes are considerably more comprehensive than those of the past, the result is still a lumped representation of

W.P. CHARETTE, A.H. KADISH AND R. SRIDHAR

the extremely complex processes of metabolism. However, we are taking a systems view-point; the first detail required for such an approach is a suitable representation for a subsystem. For example, we need to represent the relation between h_1, insulin concentration ahd the process of glycogenesis (glycogen formation) which we designate a subsystem. Even though we have a grossly lumped representation for this subsystem, it may be adequate to elucidate over-all system behavior. It is our perhaps sanguine view that if all of these subsystems, even though grossly approximated, are interconnected properly, a valid system representation will be obtained that will not be negated when investigations on a biochemical level reveal the detailed dynamics within all of the subsystems in the over-all model.

COMMENTS

A model is not very useful unless it can predict in a consistent manner the response to stimuli different from those used to determine the parameters of the model. It is evident that very little substantiation of the proposed models has been carried out in the literature by proper predictions.

Most of the models of glucose regulation seem to be concerned only with hyperglycemic states. This has the tendency to de-emphasize the effects of many hormones which play an important part in over-all glucose homeostasis.

A major shortcoming of all the models considered up to the present time appears to be that they are concerned only with short term (two to six hours) regulation problems. These models clearly cannot entirely account for the interrelating and obviously essential roles of the coupling among glucose, fat, and protein in the glucose regulation problem. As an example, we may cite the long-term effects of disturbed g lucose regulation, which are clearly coupled to deranged fat metabolism. Furthermore the variations of glucose tolerance with age and obesity, atherosclerosis, and diabetes assume great importance over time intervals of years. Such variations are undetectable over the time intervals in which the current models are meaningful. A long term metabolism model should eventually be available for better understanding of health and disease.

In the authors' opinion, one of the great difficulties in getting accurate models is the sparse reliable data that is available which is in a form useful for solving inverse problems. The solution of the inverse problem requires that data be obtained for different and pertinent types of stimuli on the same individual. It does not make sense from the modeling point of view to use glucose tolerance data from one individual and insulin response from another. Moreover, it is extremely important that the responses of interest be sampled at a rate that is consistent with the model. For example, a large number of models can be constructed which will agree very well with the response to an oral glucose load if only four data points spaced every half hour are taken. Some of these models can be completely nonsensical even from the point of view of a layman!

It is also very important to know precisely the exact times at which various stimuli were applied and the various responses were sampled. As an example of such imprecision it is common practice in the literature to begin measurement on the response to an I.V. glucose load from the end of the infusion. This results in a loss of critical information. Model parameters often have an unfortunate habit of being extremely sensitive to the instants of time at which important events take place.

We appear to have a long way to go before we can be very confident in using the mathematical models of the glucose homeostatic system for diagnostic purposes and for prescribing the suitable types of corrections in case of disease. However, we have also come a long way. The difficult first step of convincing researchers that models do have a place in understanding and alleviating disease evidently has been accomplished.

REFERENCES

1. E. Ackerman, J.W. Rosevear, W.F. McGuckin, "A Mathematical Model of the Glucose-Tolerance Test", Phys. Med. Biol. 9, No. 2, 203-213; 1964.

2. E. Ackerman, L.C. Gatewood, J.W. Rosevear, G.D. Molnar, "Model Studies of Blood-Glucose Regulation", Bull. Math. Biophysics 27, 21-36; 1965.

3. D.S. Amatuzio, et. al., "Interpretation of the Rapid Intravenous Glucose Tolerance Test in Normal Individuals and in Mild Diabetes Mellitus", J. Clin. Invest 32, 428-435; 1953.

4. R.P. Beliles, "Theoretical and Experimental Studies of Factors Affecting Blood Glucose Regulation", Ph.D. Thesis, Pharmacology, Iowa State University; 1962.

5. R.E. Bellman and R.E. Kalaba, Quasilinearization and Nonlinear Boundary-Value Problems, American Elsevier Publishing Co., New York; 1965.

6. V.W. Bolie, "Glucose-Insulin Feedback Theory", Third Int. Conf. on Med. Elec.; July 22, 1960.

7. V.W. Bolie, "Coefficients of Normal Blood Glucose Regulation", J. of Clin. Invest. 39, Part 2, 783-788; 1960.

8. E. Cerasi, "An Analog Computer Model for the Insulin Response to Glucose Infusion", Acta Endocrinologica 55, 163-183; 1967.

9. W.P. Charette, A.H. Kadish, R. Sridhar, "A Nonlinear Dynamic Model of Endocrine Control of Metabolic Processes", 7th. Int. Conf. on Med. and Biol. Eng., Stockholm; August 16, 1967.

10. S. Goldman, "Cybernetic Aspects of Homeostasis", Mineral Metabolism, Academic Press, Vol. I, Part A, Chapter 3; 1960.

11. A.H. Kadish, "Cybernetics of Blood Sugar Regulation and Servo System Disease Research", Instrumentation Methods for Predictive Medicine, Instrument Society of America, Ch. 8, pp. 87-106; 1966.

12. F.C. McLean, "The Homeostasis of Blood Sugar", Diabetes 13, No. 2, 198-202; 1964.

13. J.C. Seed, F.S. Acton, A.J. Stunkard, "A Model for the Appraisal of Glucose Metabolism", Clin. Pharm. and Therapeutics 3, No.2, 191-215; 1962.

14. D.M. Shames, "A Theoretical Study of the Blood Glucose Regulatory System", M.D. Thesis, Yale University School of Medicine, 1965.

15. L.E. Wolaver, "Mathematical Model for Blood Sugar Regulation of the Human Body and its Control in Diabetes Mellitus", AICA Congress, Lausanne, Switzerland; September 2, 1967.

16. D.E. Wrede, "Development of a Mathematical Model for a Biological Feedback System with Particular Application to Glucose Metabolism", Ph.D. Thesis, Biological Chemistry, University of Cincinnati; 1963.

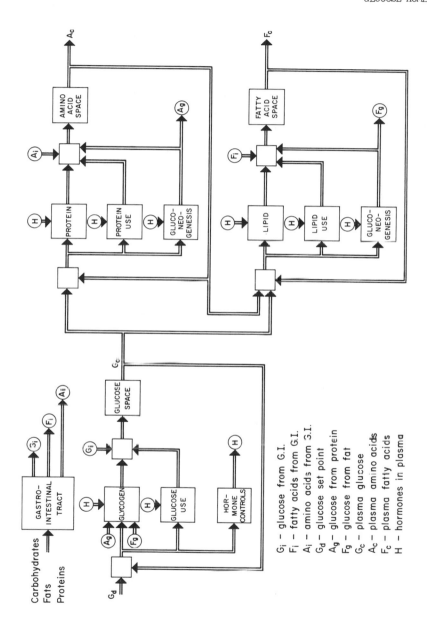

Figure 1. METABOLIC CONTROL SYSTEM

G_i – glucose from G.I.
F_i – fatty acids from G.I.
A_i – amino acids from G.I.
G_d – glucose set point
A_g – glucose from protein
F_g – glucose from fat
G_c – plasma glucose
A_c – plasma amino acids
F_c – plasma fatty acids
H – hormones in plasma

W.P. CHARETTE, A.H. KADISH AND R. SRIDHAR

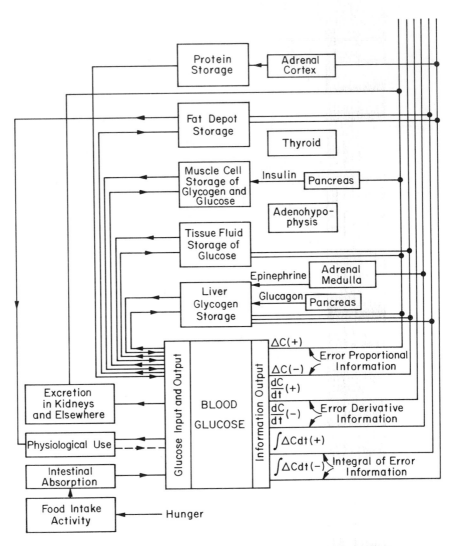

Figure 2. GOLDMAN'S PROPOSED GLUCOSE MODEL

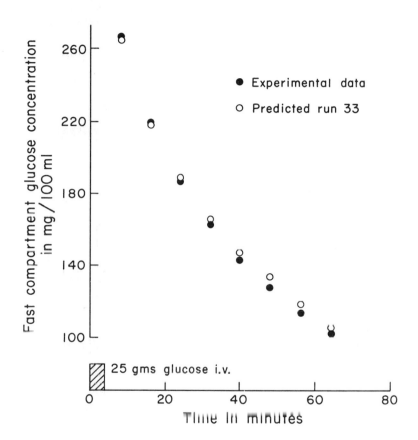

Figure 3. SEED, ACTON, STUNKARD TWO COMPARTMENT
MODEL COMPARISON WITH DATA AVERAGED
OVER 70 NORMAL SUBJECTS FROM AMATUZIO.

W.P. CHARETTE, A.H. KADISH AND R. SRIDHAR

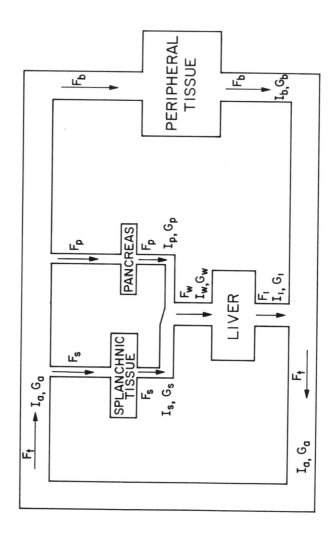

Figure 4. BELILES' FIVE COMPARTMENT GLUCOSE MODEL

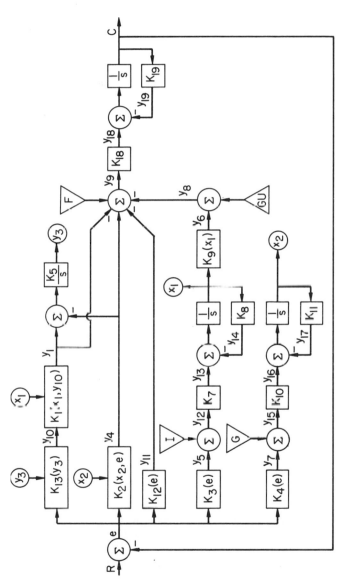

Figure 5. GLUCOSE MODEL–TWO HORMONES

W.P. CHARETTE, A.H. KADISH AND R. SRIDHAR

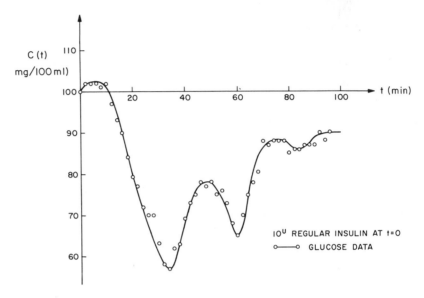

Figure 6. PLASMA GLUCOSE-SUBJECT Z 9-10-66

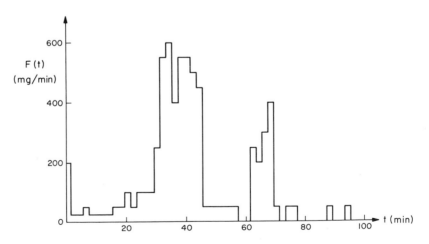

Figure 7. GLUCOSE INPUT-SUBJECT Z 9-10-66

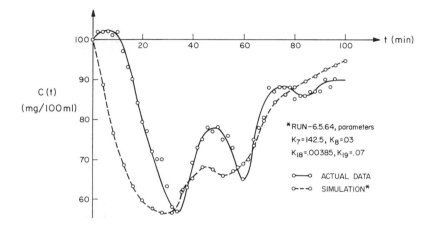

Figure 8. SIMULATION OF SUBJECT Z 9-10-66

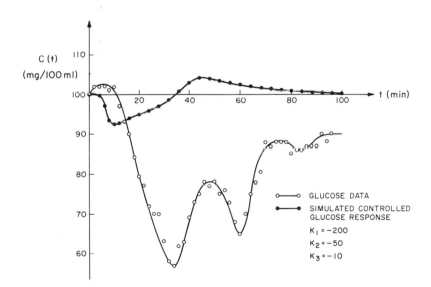

Figure 9. SIMULATED CLOSED LOOP CONTROL OF
PLASMA GLUCOSE

W.P. CHARETTE, A.H. KADISH AND R. SRIDHAR

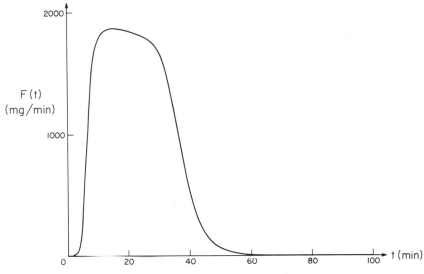

Figure 10. SIMULATED GLUCOSE CONTROL INPUT

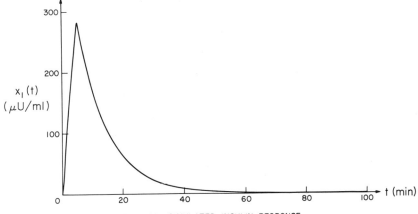

Figure 11. SIMULATED INSULIN RESPONSE

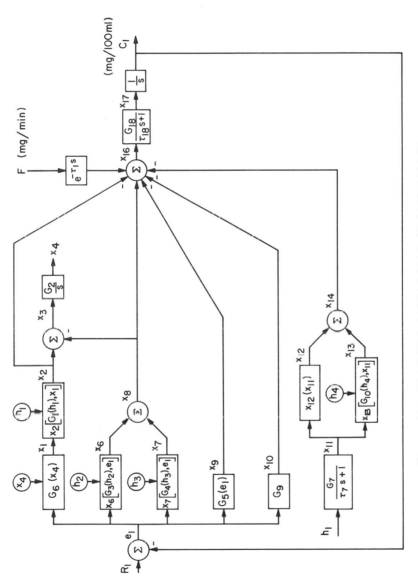

Figure 12. GLUCOSE METABOLIC PLANT MODEL

W.P. CHARETTE, A.H. KADISH AND R. SRIDHAR

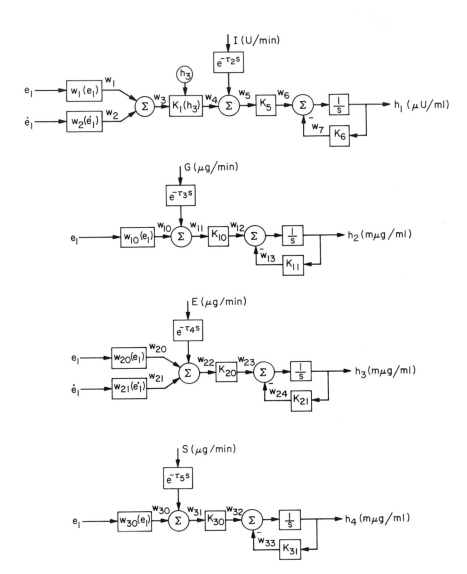

Figure 13. HORMONE CONTROLLER MODEL

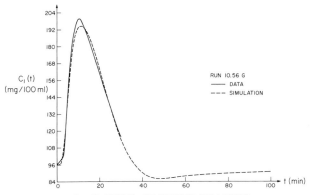

Figure 14. SUBJECT K - 15 G I.V. GLUCOSE OVER 3 MINUTES

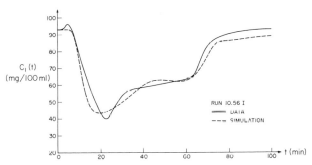

Figure 15. SUBJECT K 5ᵘ INSULIN AT T=0, I MG GLUCAGON AT T=58

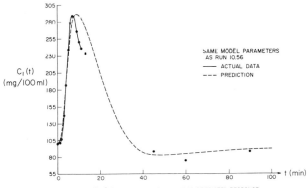

Figure 16. SUBJECT K - 30 G I.V. GLUCOSE PREDICTED RESPONSE

5. CURRENT VIEWS ON THE BEHAVIOUR OF THE THYROID-PITUITARY SYSTEM

K. BROWN-GRANT
Department of Human Anatomy, University of Oxford and Department of Physiology, Stanford University

INTRODUCTION

The title of this paper, the behaviour of the thyroid-pituitary system is intended to cover the functioning of this system in the normal state and in response to a variety of experimental stimuli (or inputs) in the intact animal. As a basis for our thinking, experimental design, and interpretation of our results, we need some theoretical model, however crude, of the system and in general the experimentalist only arrives at this by a process of physiological dissection in which initially certain features of the system are studied in isolation so far as possible. I intend to try to describe how our present views have been arrived at. The detailed evidence, and happily there is considerable agreement both as to experimental results and interpretation, may be found in several recent reviews by Bogdanove [7], Brown-Grant [9, 10], D'Angelo [12], Harris [24], Purves [35], and Reichlin [37]. It should perhaps be stressed that in much of the early work the evidence that thyrotrophin (TSH) secretion was altered was indirect, being based on measurements of changes in the activity of the thyroid gland as reflected in changes in radio-iodine metabolism. The development of more sensitive and specific bio-assay methods and of radio-immunoassays for TSH in recent years has provided the tools for the direct confirmation of many earlier assumptions.

* Supported by grants from the Lalor Foundation and the Wellcome Trust

THE THYROID-PITUITARY AXIS

Historically, the first suggestion of an interaction between the two glands was the description of pituitary enlargement in cretins by Niepce in 1851. P.E. Smith, in 1916, [41] described hypofunction of the thyroid after hypophysectomy in the tadpole and later in the rat [42]. The identification of a specific protein hormone in extracts of pituitary gland which was capable of stimulating the thyroid involved many workers but in particular the pioneering studies of H.M. Evans and his group at the University of California, Berkeley, deserve mention. The concept of a balanced, reciprocal relationship between the two glands was implied in the studies of Aron, van Caulaert and Stahl [2] in 1931. In this reciprocal relationship an excess of thyroid hormone, thyroxine [T_4 will in general be used as an abbreviation, thus conveniently ignoring, because for the most part the experimental evidence is not available, the contribution of the second thyroid gland hormone, $3-5-3^1$- triiodothyronine] depresses TSH secretion and conversely a lowered circulating T_4 level, from whatever cause, stimulates TSH secretion in an attempt to restore the *status quo*. This relationship was described in more mechanistic terms as a servo or negative feed-back system by R.G. Hoskins [27] in 1949 and this primitive model will certainly deal with a considerable proportion of the well established physiological findings related to the thyroid-pituitary system that were available at that time.

The life span of models is, however, rather short; by 1949 it was already known that an additional feature would need to be introduced for the pioneering studies of F.H.A. Marshall, of the University of Cambridge in 1942, on the role of external stimuli from the environment in the control of reproductive processes had indicated that the hypothalamic area of the brain, acting through the pituitary, influenced gonadotrophin secretion [37]. G.W. Harris, also of Cambridge, put forward the view [21, 22] that this control might be exerted by the release of neuro-humoral transmitters from the median eminence into the primary plexus of the hypothalamo-hypophysical portal vessel system and their passage to the anterior lobe of the pituitary to influence the secretion of the various trophic hormones. The new concepts and techniques of this branch of "Neuroendocrinology", though originally developed mainly in connection with research on the control of gonadotrophin secretion, have since been applied extensively to the study of the control of the other trophic hormones including TSH (see Schrieber, [43] for the historical background and Martini and Ganong, [32] for details of methodology).

The role of the hypothalamus in the control of TSH secretion was first studied by the more negative methods of hypothalamic lesions, pituitary stalk-section, and pituitary transplantation. One of the earliest papers to be published was that of

BEHAVIOUR OF THE THYROID-PITUITARY SYSTEM

Green [17] in 1951, and the many later studies are detailed in the reviews cited above. The outcome of these studies was an unexpected finding in view of what is known about the effects of similar procedures on the secretion of gonadotrophins, corticotrophin, and growth hormone. The finding was that the level of TSH secretion by the pituitary isolated from hypothalamic influences (sometimes referred to as the autonomous pituitary) was reduced below the normal level as expected, but it was sufficient to maintain a level of thyroid gland activity that was considerably greater than that seen in the hypophysectomised animal which was unexpected. More important than the absolute level of activity, however, was the further unexpected finding that TSH secretion could decrease or increase (at least to a limited extent) in a physiologically meaningful manner in response to increases or decreases in circulating thyroid hormone level. The implication of this is that the negative feed-back system is still operating and that the thyroxine 'receptors' or 'error-sensing' mechanism must, therefore, exist at the pituitary level. This was demonstrated more directly in 1956 by von Euler and Holmgren [44] who were the first to employ the technique of chronically implanted cannulae in the pituitary or hypothalamus to permit the repeated local administration of hormones in the conscious animal. They showed that a dose of thyroxine which was ineffective when given systemically would suppress TSH secretion when injected directly into the pituitary but was not effective when injected into the hypothalamus. In 1966, Reichlin [37] presented a detailed and critical review of the later experiments of this type. The existence of hypothalamic thyroxine 'receptors' is, at present, best regarded as 'not proven'.

THE ROLE OF THE HYPOTHALAMUS

Despite the description given above of regulation by the 'autonomous' pituitary, it is clear that the hypothalamus can influence the thyroid-pituitary system. Again selection of individual papers can only be arbitrary and full reviews were given in 1966 by Brown-Grant [9] and by Reichlin [37]. Harris and Woods [26] presented evidence of thyroid activation following electrical stimulation of the anterior hypothalamus in conscious rabbits and recently Averill and Salaman [3] have confirmed that circulating TSH levels are increased in such experiments. In 1964, both Andersson [1] in the goat and Reichlin [36] in the rat have demonstrated that local cooling of the anterior hypothalamus will activate the thyroid gland and local heating will abolish the response to a systemic cold stimulus. These experiments provide an elegant confirmation of the earlier work, based on hypothalamic lesions, that suggested that the C.N.S. was involved in the acute increase in thyroid activity that follows exposure to cold. Any realistic picture of the thyroid-pituitary system must, therefore, include both 'chemical control' exerted by thyroxine feed-

back at the pituitary level and a potential 'neural drive' exerted by the hypothalamus. It seems almost certain that the latter influence is indeed mediated, as
Harris suggested, by the release of a chemical agent from hypothalamic neurones into
the portal vessels to reach the pituitary directly. There is agreement as to the
name of this agent, thyrotrophin releasing factor or TRF, but not as to its chemical
nature. Until 1966, several groups engaged in the attempt to extract TRF and other
releasing factors from bovine or ovine hypothalami had indicated that it was probably
a small polypeptide [25] but more recently a highly active non-peptide agent has been
reported. The situation is at present changing rapidly and the details given in
Brown-Grant [10] are probably now outdated. More important for the present discussion are the reports that TRF activity has been detected in hypophysical portal vessel blood following hypothalamic stimulation [4, 15].

ADDITIONAL FACTORS OPERATING IN THE INTACT ANIMAL

Even a consideration of 'chemical' and 'neural' factors, however, cannot provide
an adequate idea of what will happen in the intact animal nor, unfortunately, form
the basis for model making. In real life the pituitary and the thyroid are not connected by closed pipes and we must consider the role of other organs and tissues in
altering the level of TSH and of thyroxine to which the thyroid and pituitary are
exposed. Variations in the volume of distribution and the biological half-life of
TSH may occur. So far the major change reported has been an increase in half-life
of TSH in severe hypothyroidism [5]. Under these circumstances, peripheral TSH levels no longer bear their normal relationship to production rates. At present it
appears that changes on the TSH side may be neglected, at least in acute experiments.
Changes in the peripheral metabolism of thyroxine have been more extensively studied.
The major pathways of T_4 disposal are deiodination and biliary secretion of the intact hormone or a conjugate, followed by a varying amount of entero-hepatic recircu-
lation and eventual loss in the faeces. Studies of thyroxine metabolism should,
ideally, be part of any experimental investigation of changes in the thyroid-pituitary system and these factors must be included in any model. A less immediately
obvious complication arises from the physico-chemical state of the thyroid hormone
in the blood. Two examples may help to illustrate this; both were initially thought
to be in conflict with the concept of a simple negative feed-back control of TSH
(Brown-Grant, [11]). Following oestrogen administration or during pregnancy in the
human the circulating thyroid hormone level is raised to a level that in a normal
individual would give rise to clinical signs of hyperthyroidism. However there is
no evidence of this and despite the *raised* hormone level, the activity of the thyroid

BEHAVIOUR OF THE THYROID-PITUITARY SYSTEM

gland is *normal or even increased*. The second example is the rat treated with
dinitrophenol (DNP) or drugs of the salicylate group; here the situation is reversed
and a *reduced* circulating hormone level is found *without* any evidence of thyroid
activation. The explanation of these paradoxes is that, in plasma, thyroxine is
reversibly bound by non-covalent linkages to a specific protein or proteins with a
high affinity for the hormone——the thyroxine binding protein(s) or TBP. Current
estimates for the human suggest that only about 0.05% of the total plasma thyroxine
is present in the free or unbound state but that the effects on the peripheral tissues, the rate of hormone degradation, and the feed-back influence on the pituitary
are related to the free fraction rather than the total thyroxine content of plasma.
The effect of oestrogen is to increase the plasma concentration of one of the binding proteins in the human, TBG; the same *free* T_4 content is now achieved only at a
higher *total* T_4 level. Transient changes in thyroid activity and in the rate of
T_4 disposal achieve a readjustment to this new level and the apparent paradox is
resolved if we consider free rather than total thyroxine as the controlled variable.
The effect of DNP or salicylate is more complex; it appears to compete with thyroxine for the binding sites on TBP. Effectively, this results in lowering of the
number of sites available to T_4, the equivalent of a lowering of TBP levels. The
result is that the same free T_4 concentration is achieved at a lower total concentration and again the anomalous situation of a normal level of thyroid gland activity in the presence of a reduced level of thyroid hormone in the blood is resolved.
The original review of Robbins and Rall [40] in 1960 is still the best starting
point for further study of the role of binding proteins; two recent studies by Good,
Hetzel and Hogg [16] in 1965 and by Reichlin and Utiger [38] in 1967 provide direct
experimental support for these ideas.

AN ANALYSIS OF THE SYSTEM RESPONSE TO COLD EXPOSURE

With the three factors of chemical control, neural drive, and changes in peripheral tissues in mind, the effects of a classic stimulus to the thyroid-pituitary
system, exposure to cold, can now be considered. In an earlier section some of the
evidence that the hypothalamus (probably by the release of TRF) was involved in the
acute response to cold (over a period of perhaps eight hours) was reviewed. Lesion
of the anterior hypothalamus or transplanation of the pituitary block this response
and it can be induced by local cooling of the anterior hypothalamus despite a rise
in general body temperature. When exposure to cold is more prolonged (a period of
days or weeks), there are persistent reports that such lesions or pituitary stalk-
section do not abolish the response. The explanation appears to be that prolonged

exposure to cold results in an increased rate of T_4 disposal by a variety of mechanisms, principally as a consequence of increased food intake, increased faecal mass, and hence increased loss of T_4 by the biliary-faecal pathway in the rat. Increased deiodination of T_4 by the peripheral tissues under the influence of catecholamines may also be involved. The more rapid turnover of T_4 results in lowered blood levels during chronic exposure to cold: the feed-back mechanism can operate, as we know, at the pituitary level and probably accounts for the response seen in lesioned or stalk-sectioned animals chronically exposed to cold. Panda and Turner [34] have recently (1967) presented direct evidence of raised plasma TSH levels in lesioned rats after 3 days exposure to a temperature of 4°C. In 1966, Koch, Jobin and Fortier [30] also provided evidence of lowered T_4 levels in *intact* rats exposed to cold for long periods. It is an interesting point, both for the biologist and the engineer, that there may be a persistent error in the feed-back system under these conditions. It is also apparent that the so-called hypothalamic 'thyrostat' is not reset to provide a higher T_4 level during prolonged cold exposure. Indeed the initial period of raised T_4 level and thyroid hyperactivity is quite transient as may be seen from the original figures reproduced in the 1966 review by Reichlin [37] and frequently a fall towards control values begins before the end of even quite brief periods of exposure to cold. The chronic thyroid response to cold exposure can be prevented by T_4 administration as was demonstrated in the classic experiments of Dempsey and Astwood [13]. The acute response can also be blocked by T_4 as was shown for the hamster by Knigge [29] in 1960 and for the goat by Andersson [1] in 1964. The falling off in the response after the first few hours of acute cold exposure may be due to the high endogenous T_4 level. A rather similar failure to maintain an initial raised T_4 level is seen in many stimulation experiments (see figures reproduced by and those in the original papers cited in the 1966 review by Reichlin [37], and there are no published reports known to me in which electrical stimulation of the hypothalamus has been shown to be capable of producing a sustained rise in circulating T_4 level. If we accept that the initial rise in acute cold exposure or after electrical stimulation is due to release of TRF, then the spontaneous falling off or the blockade of the response by T_4 could be due to either a "feed-back" effect at the hypothalamic level preventing TRF release or at the pituitary level preventing the response to TRF. The second explanation seems more likely to me as there is evidence that the action of exogenous materials with TRF activity is reduced or abolished by T_4 administration (see the recent paper by Bowers et al. [8] for references).

BEHAVIOUR OF THE THYROID-PITUITARY SYSTEM

PROBLEMS ARISING FROM THIS ANALYSIS

If the view given in the preceding section is correct, it raises serious difficulties for any theory or model that assumes that the hypothalamus tonically stimulates the pituitary with respect to TSH secretion and sets the level of thyroid
gland activity. If we attempt to make a block diagram of such a system we find first
that the evidence for an error detector (feed-back of T_4 at the hypothalamic level
to regulate TRF discharge) is, on the whole, unconvincing. Secondly, we are now
faced with the problem that the effectiveness of TRF as a driving mechanism is altered by changes in circulating T_4 level, which we regard as the variable under control. How can the hypothalamus act as part of the homeostatic mechanism when it is
not apparently monitoring the controlled variable and when the effector mechanism
can be blocked? The difficulty may be more apparent than real and criticisms from
both biologists and engineers are expected. However, if the problem is not resolved,
then perhaps a rather modified block diagram is more appropriate in which the hypothalamus figures as a source of a disturbance signal, no more and no less important
for the operation of the regulatory system than an injection of exogenous TSH or T_4.

This in turn raises several problems. Principally, if the hypothalamus is not
tonically driving the pituitary, then why is the level of thyroid activity reduced by
lesions, stalk-section, or transplanation of the pituitary as the vast majority of
investigators agree it is? One reason may be that the T_4 disposal rate (the load on
the system) is reduced; the procedures described are really rather drastic and many
other endocrine and somatic systems are also affected. Lower consumption of T_4 means
a lower required output from the gland, hence the hypoactivity; the reduced load
theory, with its implication that the animals are not really hypothyroid at all, is
consistent with the finding that the thyroid-pituitary system can operate at higher
levels if called upon to do so. Measurements of T_4 levels and studies of T_4 metabolism have only rarely been carried out in such animals. A recent paper (1967) by
Halasz, Florsheim, Corcoran and Gorski [20] is an exception. Their study concerned
thyroid function in animals subjected to hypothalamic deafferentation by means of
the Halász knife and they report reduced PBI levels. But even reduced PBI levels
are not conclusive evidence of hypothyroidism as we have seen in the discussion of
the role of binding proteins. Until the free T_4 levels are measured, the 'reduced
load' hypothesis, plus changes in TBP, remains a possible explanation of these findings. A second difficulty with the assumption that there is no tonic secretion of
TRF concerns the acute response to "stress". An acute decrease in TSH secretion in
"stressed" animals was suggested on indirect grounds in 1955 (see Harris [23]), and
has now been confirmed in several laboratories by direct measurement (see Ducommun,

Sakiz and Guillemin, [14] for references). Cessation of TRF secretion could account
for these findings, but if this is not normally secreted, some other mechanisms must
be sought. The idea that CRF simultaneously stimulates ACTH and depresses TSH secretion is not born out by the results of Ducommun et al but their experimental design did not exclude the possibility that CRF secretion continued with its effect on
ACTH release being blocked by Dexamethasone but not its action on the pituitary to
suppress TSH secretion [14]. Less acute changes in TSH secretion in response to
stress may involve alterations in TBP and free T_4 levels and operate through the
'chemical' feed-back mechanism (Haibach and McKenzie, [19]).

DISCUSSION

Many questions remain to be answered about the thyroid-pituitary system. Some
of the necessary investigations are immediately obvious to any biologist, the chemical nature of TRF in the hypothalamus and in portal vessel blood, for instance.
The biochemical mechanism by which T_4 exerts its negative "feed-back" effect on pituitary TSH secretion is another. It seems improbable that a simple exposure of the
thyrotrophs to a given concentration of T_4, probably proportional to the free T_4
fraction of the plasma hormone content, is all that is involved. There is some support for the view that the rate of deiodination (possibly mono-deiodination) of T_4
by pituitary tissue may provide the immediate signal to which the thyrotrophs respond (Mouriz, Morreale de Escobar and Escobar del Rey, [33] though the most pertinent direct attack on this problem did not entirely support this view (Reichlin,
Volpert and Werner, [39]). It should be noted also that the work so far has been
confined to the rat and that an extension to other species is desirable. There are
many other questions, however, that are not quite so obvious until, as Grodins pointed out, one begins to think in terms of control system theory, in even the most sim-
ple-minded way, and attempts to write block diagrams, however elementary [18]. The
most critical question, it seems to me, is whether the hypothalamus does or can drive
the thyroid-pituitary system chronically. The necessary experimental design to answer this question may involve a much more rigorous application of control system
theory and the recent work of Stear and DiStefano which is presented in this volume
illustrates this and shows how experiments that a biologist would not normally under-
take may help to resolve his problems.

In summary, the thyroid-pituitary system is a complex and rapidly responding
one. We already know that such diverse factors as (1) hormonal feed-back (chemical
or humoral control) at the pituitary level, (2) acute, and possibly chronic, neural
drive from the hypothalamus, (3) variations in peripheral TSH and T_4 distribution

BEHAVIOUR OF THE THYROID-PITUITARY SYSTEM

and metabolism, and (4) variations in the binding of T_4 to specific plasma proteins must be included in our theoretical considerations and our experimental investigation of the behaviour of the system in the intact animal. Clearly no simple mathematical model of such a complex system is possible and, if the biologist is to benefit from the application of control systems theory to his problems, he requires both theoretical guidance and practical assistance from those expert in this field.

Indeed the biologist may eventually ask more of the systems analyst than the physical scientist because of the inescapably non-linear nature of living control systems. Too many of the texts addressed to biologists are still mainly concerned with the transfer function approach to the analysis of linear systems which has been so successful in engineering practice. There are signs that this problem has been recognized, however. A recent book (1966), Bayliss [6] writing as a biologist, introduces non-linear systems in some detail at an early stage. From the other side, Iberall & Cardon [28] pinpoint the need "to attempt to steer him (the biologist) away from too easy acceptance of elementary control theory." But until the two sides can be brought together to explore the possibilities and define the areas most likely to yield useful results, little will be achieved.

I would like to express my personal thanks to the organisors and sponsors for the opportunity to attend this Conference and to take part in just such an interchange of ideas and information both by formal presentations in public and by informal discussions in private.

REFERENCES

1. Anderson, B. (1964). Hypothalamic temperature and thyroid activity. *Ciba Foundation Study Group*, 18, 35-50.

2. Aron, M., Van Caulaert, C. & Stahl, J. (1931), L'equilibre entre l'hormone prehypophysaire et l'hormone throidienne dans le milieu interieur à l'état normal et à l'état pathologique. *Comp. Rend. Soc. Biol.* (Paris) 107, 64-66.

3. Averill, R.L.W., & Salaman, D.F. (1967) Elevation of plasma thyrotrophin TSH) during electrical stimulation in the rabbit hypothalamus. *Endocrinology*, 81, 173-178.

4. Averill, R.L.W., Salaman, D.F., & Worthington, W.D. (1966). Thyrotrophin releasing factor in hypophyseal portal blood. *Nature* (Lond.) 211, 144-45.

5. Bakke, J.L. & Lawrence, N.L. (1962). Disappearance rate and distribution of exogenous thyrotropin in the rat. *Endocrinology* 71, 43-56.

6. Bayliss, L.E. (1966). Living Control Systems. London: English Universities Press.

7. Bogdanove, E.M. (1962). Regulation of TSH Secretion. *Federation Proc.* 21, 623-627.

8. Boyers, C.V., Schally, A.V., Reynolds, G.A. & Hawley, W.D. (1967). Interactions of L-thyroxine or L-triiodothyronine and thyrotropin releasing factor on the release and synthesis of thyrotropin from the anterior pituitary gland of mice. *Endocrinology*, 81, 741-747.

9. Brown-Grant, K. (1966). The control of TSH secretion. Chap. 7, pp. 235-269. In *The Pituitary Gland*. Ed. G.W. Harris & B.T. Donovan. Vol. 2. London: Butterworths.

10. Brown-Grant, K. (1967A). The control of thyroid secretion. *Journal of Clinical Pathology*. Symposium on the Thyroid Gland. pp. 327-332.

11. Brown-Grant, K. (1967B). Regulation and control in the endocrine system. Chap. 8, pp. 176-255. In *Regulation and Control in Living Systems*. Ed. H. Kalmus. London: Wiley.

12. D'Angelo, S.A. (1963). Central nervous regulation of the secretion and release of thyroid stimulating hormone. Chap. 6. pp. 158-205. In *Advances in Neuro-endocrinology*. Ed. A. Nalbandov. Urbana: University of Illinois Press.

13. Dempsey, E.W. & Astwood, E.B. (1943). Determination of the rate of thyroid hormone secretion at various environmental temperatures. *Endocrinology*, 32, 509-518.

14. Ducommun, P., Sakiz, E., & Guillemin, R. (1966). Dissocation of the acute secretions of thyrotropin and adrenocorticotropin. *Amer. J. Physiol.* 210, 1257-1259.

15. Good, B.F. (1967). Personal Communication.

16. Good, B.F., Hetzel, B.S. & Hogg, B.M. (1965). Studies of the control of thyroid function in rats: effects of salicylate and related drugs. *Endocrinology*, 77, 674-682.

17. Greer, M.A. (1951). Evidence of hypothalamic control of pituitary release of thyrotropin. *Proc. Soc. Exp. Biol. Med.* 77, 603-608.

18. Grodins, F.S. (1963). Control theory and biological systems. London: Columbia University Press.

19. Haibach, H. & McKenzie, J.M. (1967). Increased free thyroxine postoperatively in the rat. *Endocrinology*, 81, 435-439.

20. Halasz, D., Florsheim, W.H., Corcoran, N.L. & Gorski, R.A. (1967). Thyro-trophic hormone secretion in rats after partial or total interruption of neural afferents to the medial basal hypothalamus. *Endocrinology*, 80, 1075-1082.

21. Harris, G.W. (1948). Neural control of the pituitary gland. *Physiol. Rev.* 28, 139-179.

22. Harris, G.W. (1955A). Neural control of the pituitary gland. *Monographs of the Physiological Society*, 3. London: Arnold.

23. Harris, G.W. (1955B). The reciprocal relationship between the thyroid and adrenocortical responses to stress. *Ciba Foundation Colloquia on Endocrinology*, 8, 531-550.

24. Harris, G.W. (1964). A summary of some recent research on brain-thyroid relationships. *Ciba Foundation Study Group*, 18, 3-16.

25. Harris, G.W., Reed, M. & Fawcett, C.P. (1966). Hypothalamic releasing factors and the control of anterior pituitary function. *Brit. Med. Bull.* 22, 266-272.

BEHAVIOUR OF THE THYROID-PITUITARY SYSTEM

26. Harris, G.W. & Woods, J.W. (1958). The effect of electrical stimulation of the hypothalamus or pituitary gland on thyroid activity. *J. Physiol.* 143, 246-274.

27. Hoskins, R.G. (1949). The thyroid-pituitary apparatus as a servo (feed-back) mechanism. *J. Clin. Endocr.* 9, 1429-1431.

28. Iberall, A.S. & Cardon, S.Z. (1965). Regulation and control in biological systems. Proceedings of the IFAC Tokyo Symposium on Systems Engineering for Control Systems Design. pp. 436-473.

29. Knigge, K.M. (1960). Time study of acute cold-induced acceleration of thyroidal I^{131} release in the hamster. *Proc. Soc. Exp. Med.* 104, 368-371.

30. Koch, B., Jobin, M. & Fortier, C. (166). TSH and thyroxine secretion rates following prolonged exposure to cold in the rat. *Federation Proc.* 25, 516 (Abstract).

31. Marshall, F.H.A. (1942). Exteroceptive factors in sexual periodicity. *Biol. Rev. Cambridge Phil. Soc.* 17, 68-89.

32. Martini, L., & Ganong, W.F. (Ed.) (1966). Neuroendocrinology, Vol. 1. New York: Academic Press.

33. Mouriz, J., Morreale de Escobar, G., & Escobar del Rey, F. (1966). Evaluation of the peripheral deiodination of L-thyroxine as an index of its thyrotrophin suppressing effectiveness. *Endocrinology,* 79, 248-260.

34. Panda, J.N. & Turner, C.W. (1967). Hypothalamic control of thyrotrophin secretion. *J. Physiol.* 192, 1-12.

35. Purves, H.D. (1964). Control of thyroid function. Chap. 1. pp. 1-38. In *The Thyroid Gland.* Ed. R. Pitt-Rivers and W.R. Trotter. Vol. 2. London: Butterworths.

36. Reichlin, S. (1964). Function of the hypothalamus in regulation of pituitary-thyroid activity. *Ciba Foundation Study Group,* 18, 17-32.

37. Reichlin, S. (1966). Control of thyrotropic hormone secretion. Chap. 12, pp. 445-536. In *Neuroendocrinology,* Vol. 1. Ed. Martini, L. and Ganong, W.F. New York: Academic Press.

38. Reichlin, S. & Utiger, R.D. (1967). Regulation of the pituitary-thyroid axis in man: relationship of TSH concentration to concentration of free and total thyroxine in plasma. *J. Clin. Endocr.* 27, 251-255.

39. Reichlin, S., Volpert, E.M. & Werner, S.C. (1966). Hypothalamic influence on thyroxine monodeiodination by rat anterior pituitary gland. *Endocrinology,* 78, 302-306.

40. Robbins, J. & Rall, J.E. (1960). Proteins associated with the thyroid hormones. *Physiol. Rev.* 40, 415-489.

41. Smith, P.E. (1916). Experimental ablation of the hypophysis in the frog embryo. *Science,* 44, 280-282.

42. Smith, P.E. (1927). The disabilities caused by hypophysectomy and their repair. The tuberal (hypothalamic) syndrome in the rat. *J. Amer. Med. Assoc.* 88, 158-161.

43. Schreiber, V. (1963). The hypothalamo-hypophysial system. Prague:Czechoslovak Academy of Sciences.

44. von Euler, C. & Holmgren, B.C. (1956). The thyroxine "receptor" of the thyroid-pituitary system. *J. Physiol.* 131, 125-136.

6. MODELING AND CONTROL ASPECTS OF THYROID FUNCTION

JOSEPH J. DISTEFANO III AND EDWIN B. STEAR**
Department of Engineering, University of California, Los Angeles, Los Angeles, California

---

INTRODUCTION

One of the most firmly established results of a vast amount of research dating back to the very origins of physiology is that the two major systems involved in the control of all important physiological variables and processes are the central nervous system and the endocrine systems. In more recent times, it has been further established that these two types of systems often act jointly to exercise this control. This important discovery has led to the development of the new field of neuroendocrinology which is directly concerned with the interrelationships between the central nervous system and the endocrine systems. One example in which both the central nervous system and an endocrine system act jointly to exercise control of physiological variables and processes is the control of plasma thyroid hormone levels. This particular case has been extensively investigated and it constitutes the subject matter of the present paper.

This paper has three related objectives. The first is to examine models and modeling from several points of view in order to sketch the spectrum of possible models. This will provide some perspective from which to view models of neuroendocrine systems in general and the particular models of thyroid function to be discussed later. The second objective is to provide a current review of known models of the regulation and control aspects of thyroid function in order to indicate the current status of research in this area. The final objective is to indicate some of the inadequacies of the models reviewed and to show, by means of a specific example, how such inadequacies can usually be overcome at the expense

---
*   The preparation of this paper and the research on which it is based was supported in part by NASA Grant NsG 237-62 and a grant from the National Science Foundation.
**   The authors are Assistant Professor of Engineering and Associate Professor of Engineering, respectively, and are regular faculty members of the Information Systems Division.

JOSEPH J. DISTEFANO III AND EDWIN B. STEAR

of further complication and sophistication of the models. These objectives are
pursued, in turn, in the next three sections of the paper.

SOME ASPECTS OF MODELS AND MODELING

Because the word "model" can be properly used to refer to any one of wide
variety of things (e.g., a woman who wears somebody elses' clothes for pay; a
scaled down, geometrically congruent likeness of a physical object; a mathematical
description of certain features of a system or object), it is important to clarify
one's use of the word at the outset of any discussion in which the word is used
in a specific manner. In this paper, the word "model" will be used to refer to
any set of mathematical expressions used to describe the interrelationships
between a set of variables, some or all of which are identified in a one-to-one
fashion with measurable attributes or aspects of some real-world system or object,
or classes of such systems or objects*. This use of the word is rather commonly
accepted by physiologists, endocrinologists, engineer's, mathematicians, etc. who
are interested in "models and modeling" of biological systems. In the case of
physiological systems in general and endocrine systems in particular, the models
usually consist of sets of algebraic equations and/or differential equations, or
differential-difference equations, if appropriate. However, other possibilities
exist and are sometimes used effectively as will be apparent from some of the subsequent discussion.

Probably the single most important factor which ultimately determines the
general characteristics of any given model of a system is the use to which the model
is to be put. In this regard, at least three different uses can be distinguished;
namely, (1) to efficiently summarize and express the currently available scientific
knowledge of some well-defined system or class of systems (this use has been called
"bookeeping" by F.E. Yates), (2) as a tool to help formulate meaningful new scientific experiments on a system and, in most cases, to predict the results of such experiments, and (3) to predict particular specific responses of a system due to well-
defined inputs or stimulation such as might occur in a clinical setting.

A second important factor which determines the general characteristics of any
given model is the type of mathematical expressions of which it is composed. The
simplest type of mathematical expression which can be used to develop a model is an
ordinary algebraic relationship or equation. Sets of algebraic equations are used

---

*   Only deterministic models are considered in this paper.

to express static and/or steady-state* relationships between model variables; i.e., are used as models of static and/or steady-state aspects of real systems. If $x_1, \ldots, x_n$ are used denote the (internal) model variables and if $u_1, \ldots, u_m$ are used to denote external or exogenous inputs to the model, then these models are of the generic form

$$f_i(x_1,\ldots,x_n, u_1,\ldots,u_m) = 0 \quad , \quad i = 1,\ldots,k \qquad (1)$$

where not necessarily all of the x_j and u_e appear in each of the equations. The number of independent equations in the set (i.e., k) is indicative of the comprehensiveness and/or level of detail of the model. Such models can be either qualitative or quantitative depending on how well the functions $f_i(\cdot)$ are known. Often only some very general characteristics of the $f_i(\cdot)$ are known from experimental results (e.g., if it is known only that $f_i(\cdot)$ is a function of x_j and that $f_i(\cdot)$ increases when x_j increases). However, even in this case such models are useful for describing the steady-state behaviour of systems.

Most often the forms of the functions $f_i(\cdot)$ are known in parametric form; i.e., Eqs. (1) are of the form

$$f_i(x_1,\ldots,x_n, u_1,\ldots,u_m, p_1,\ldots,p_k) = 0 \qquad (2)$$

In this case the functions $f_i(\cdot)$ and, hence, the model become completely quantitative once the parameters $p_1,p_2,\ldots,p_k$ are specified. Such models are usually referred to as parametric models and further experimentation on the real systems being modeled is used simply to estimate or refine estimates of the values of the parameters. The estimates of the parameters from experimental data are usually determined by least squares curve fitting or linear or nonlinear regression [18] depending on whether the functions $f_i(\cdot)$ are linear or nonlinear. The parametric representations of the functions $f_i(\cdot)$ may be chosen on the basis of previous experimental results and knowledge of the system, can be assumed in simple form on a trial basis and tested to see if they can reasonably fit the experimental data by proper choice of the parameters (e.g., linear models), or are known in form because the processes being modeled are known to satisfy well-established physico-chemical laws which can be described in parametric form (e.g., known types of enzyme kinetics).

The simplest type of mathematical expression used to develop dynamic models is an ordinary differential equation. Sets of ordinary differential equations in the model variables of the general form

$$\frac{dx_1}{dt} = f_1(x_1,\ldots,x_n, u_1,\ldots,u_m,t); \quad i = 1,\ldots,n \qquad (3)$$

*We limit our discussion of steady-states here to constant, nonperiodic steady-states. There exist many systems (e.g., the ovarian hormone control system) which exhibit periodic steady-state behavior.

JOSEPH J. DISTEFANO III AND EDWIN B. STEAR

are used to express dynamic relationships between the internal model variables, x_i, and the external or exogenous inputs, u_j. Examples of such models are contained in later sections of this paper. For a complete dynamic model one needs a differential equation for each internal model variable. However, if one is only interested in variable changes occurring with some time scale, T, (i.e., variables whose significant changes in response to inputs or changes in initial conditions characteristically occur over time intervals near T), then the internal model variables can be usefully divided into three classes as follows. First there are those internal variables whose significant changes characteristically occur over intervals of duration much larger than T. These variables can be assumed constant over intervals near T in duration and the differential equations for them can be replaced by expressions of the form

$$x_i = \text{constant} \tag{4}$$

Secondly, there are those internal variables whose significant changes characteristically occur over intervals of duration much smaller than T. These variables can be assumed to be at steady-state and the differential equations for them can be replaced by steady-state relationships of the form given in Eq. (1); i.e., it can be assumed that

$$f_i(x_1,..,x_n, u_1,...,u_m,t) = 0 \tag{5}$$

for all values of the x_i and u_j. Finally, there are the remaining internal variables whose changes are governed by differential equations of the form given in Eq. (3). It is clear that such a division of internal variables greatly simplifies the dynamic model because it reduces the number of differential equations in the model compared to a complete dynamic model. However, it does produce a model which is valid only for the time scale for which it was developed and, hence, provides a more restrictive model of the real system being modeled. As in the case of static models, dynamic models can either be qualitative or quantitative depending on how well the functions $f_i(\cdot)$ in Eq. (3) are known. Also, as in the case of static models, the $f_i(\cdot)$ are most often known or given in parametric form for the same reasons as for static models.

Relatively efficient techniques based on quasilinearization with least squares curve filtering and on nonlinear filtering of various kinds have recently become available for estimating the parameters of parametric dynamic models from dynamic response data on the real system being modeled (see, for example, [12]). In some cases, the functions $f_i(\cdot)$, or their parameters if the models are parametric, can be determined from steady-state experimental data from the real system, as illustrated in later sections of this paper. However, it should be noted that this is not always possible as is illustrated by the example of systems with rate feedback in which it is not possible to obtain the steady-state variations in the internal model variables required to estimate multiplicative parameters from steady-state experimental data.

When the real system being modeled contains signal propagation delays of the same order of magnitude as the time scale used for the dynamic model of the system, it is necessary to use <u>differential-difference equations</u> of the form

$$\frac{dx_1(t)}{dt} = f_1(x_1(t - \tau_{11}),\ldots,x_n(t - \tau_{in}),\ u_1(t),\ldots,u_m(t),t);$$

$$i = 1,\ldots,n$$

(6)

to model the real system instead of ordinary differential equations of the form given in Eq. (3). In physiological systems the common sources of such time delays are neural signal propagation delay along axons and normal circulation delays encounted by blood aliquots traveling from one organ to another through the circulatory system [19]. As before, the models can be either qualitative or quantitative depending on how well the functions $f_1(\cdot)$ and the time delays τ_{ij} are known. Also, as before, most models of this type actually in use are parametric and techniques similar to those available for dynamic models in the form of ordinary differential equations can be adapted for use to estimate the parameters from experimental dynamic response data from the real system. Usually estimates of the time delays for differential-difference equation models are estimated from more or less direct measurements of these delays in the real system.

Finally, partial differential equations are sometimes proposed for use in developing models of physiological systems [11]. However, these models are very complex and difficult to use effectively and they will not be discussed further in this paper.

In contrast to parametric dynamic models based on use of differential equations or differential-difference equations as given in Eq. (3) and Eq. (6), respectively, it is possible to develop nonparametric input-output models based on the notion of

JOSEPH J. DISTEFANO III AND EDWIN B. STEAR

system weighting function or its frequency domain equivalent, the system frequency response function. The models use mathematical expressions of the form*

$$x_i(t) = \int_0^\infty W_{ij}(\tau)u_j(t-\tau)d\tau \tag{7}$$

or

$$\bar{X}_i(j\omega) = G_{ij}(j\omega)\, \bar{U}_j(j\omega) \tag{8}$$

where $\bar{X}(j\omega)$ and $\bar{U}(j\omega)$ are the (complex) amplitudes of the harmonic components of $x_i(t)$ and $u_j(t)$, respectively. The mathematical expression given in Eq. (7) is actually a convolution integral and, of course, Eq. (8) is just an algebraic equation. However, in more recent times it has become fashionable to refer to them as linear operators on function spaces [10]. Models of the form given in Eqs. (7) and (8) were the chief types of models used by control engineers up to the mid to late 1950's, at which time they started using state-variable models of the form given by Eqs. (6) and (7). Models of the form given by Eqs. (7) and (8) have often been criticized by people interested in modeling of physiological systems because these models are linear, whereas it is claimed by these same people that physiological systems are inherently nonlinear and that understanding the nonlinear effects is essential to understanding the dynamics of the physiological system being modeled. What is apparently not realized by many of these people is that Eq. (7) (and its counterpart Eq. (8)) is just a special case of nonlinear models based on the notion of functional power series which are of the general form

---

*   Such models can be used to express the dynamic relationship between two internal model variables also in which case it would be of the form

$$x_i(t) = \int_0^\infty W_{ij}(\tau)\, x_j(t-\tau)d\tau$$

$$x_i(t) = g_i(t) + \int_0^\infty W_{ij}^1(\tau)\, u_j(t-\tau)d\tau$$

$$+ \int_0^\infty d\tau_1 \int_0^\infty d\tau_2\, W_{ij}^2\,(\tau_1,\tau_2)\, u_j(t-\tau_1)\, u_j(t-\tau_2)$$

$$+ \dots + \int_0^\infty d\tau_1 \dots \int_0^\infty d\tau_n W_{ij}^n(\tau_1,\dots,\tau_n)[u_j(t-\tau_1)\dots u_j(t-\tau_n)]$$

$$+ \dots \tag{9}$$

Hence, the natural generalization of Eq. (7) to use in modeling nonlinear systems is that given by Eq. (9). Some limited application to physiological systems of nonlinear models of the form given in Eq. (9) has already been made [17], but the difficulty in determining the $W_{ij}^k(\tau)$ severely limited the use of nonlinear models of this type. Recently a new approach to determining the $W_{ij}^k(\tau)$ from input-output data on the real system has been developed [10]. This approach uses least-squares curve fitting and a steepest-descent computing algorithm to determine the $W_{ij}^k(\tau)$. It should be noted that this approach can be used in the linear (Eq. (7)) as well as the nonlinear (Eq. (9)) case.

The advantage of models of the form given by Eq. (7) or Eq. (9) is that they express the dynamic relationship between the two model variables of interest without introducing any other variables into the model. In cases where one is only interested in particular dynamic relationships between variables two at a time for a few pairs of variables, the use of such models might be quite acceptable and might very well be more efficient computationally than the use of models of the form given in Eqs. (6) or (7). An example of where this might be expected to occur is in a clinical setting where one might be interested in predicting the response of a patient to the administration of certain quantities of exogenous inputs of therapeutic chemicals. Also, sometimes models of the form given by Eqs. (7), (8) and (9) can be used as interim models which are used to ultimately develop models of the form given by Eqs. (3) or (6) [13]. In this case, $W(\tau)$ or $G(j\omega)$ is curve fitted by a particular parametric mathematical expressions which correspond in a one-to-one manner with particular forms of the $f_i(\cdot)$ which occur in models of the form given by Eqs. (3) and (6).

JOSEPH J. DISTEFANO III AND EDWIN B. STEAR

On the other hand, models of the form given by Eqs. (7), (8), and (9) have
a related major disadvantage which has greatly limited their general use as models
of physiological systems. This disadvantage stems from the fact that, while they
do provide a quantitative model of the dynamic relationship between two variables,
they are strictly black-box, input-output models and, hence, give absolutely no
direct information concerning the details of how the output variable is related to
the input variable in the real system being modeled. That is, there is no direct
indication of how many significant intermediate variables are present in the real
system of how these intermediate variables are interrelated, or of what (if any)
physiologically relevant parameters are involved in these interrelationships. This
is in stark contrast to state-variable dynamic models of the form given by Eqs. (3)
and (6) in which all dynamically relevant variables for the time scale of interest
appear explicitly and in which the parameters appearing explicitly in the $f_i(\cdot)$ can
usually be interpreted directly in physiologically meaningful terms. Because most
of the people who are interested in modeling of physiological systems are interested
in all aspects of the system being modeled and are not just interested in modeling
the dynamic relationship between a few selected pairs of system variables, it is
clear why the thrust in physiological system modeling is almost exclusively based
on use of models of the form given in Eqs. (3) and (6).

Finally, it should be noted that while models of physiological systems of the
type discussed above can be used to represent the static or dynamic aspects of
these systems, they are not, in themselves, models of the regulation and control
aspects of the real systems being modeled. In order to obtain models of the regulation and control aspects of systems, it is necessary to identify (by some means)
which variables are the controlled or regulated variables and which are the controlling variables. When this is done, the system will be divided into two parts consisting of the plant or controlled system (whose outputs are the controlled variables
and whose inputs are the control variables) and a feedback controller (whose input
is the controlled variables and whose output is the control variables). Thus, models
of regulated or controlled systems are actually special, more sophisticated types of
models than the general types of models discussed in previous paragraphs in which
the internal and external model variables are identified in particular and meaningful ways and, as such, they express or contain even more information about a system
(especially about its structure and function) than do the more general models discussed in previous paragraphs. This is illustrated in the remaining sections of this
paper which is devoted to a discussion of regulation and control models of thyroid
function.

A REVIEW OF CONTROL AND REGULATOR MODELS OF THYROID FUNCTION

The endocrine subsystem responsible for the regulation of the amount of thyroid hormone (TH) circulating in the bloodstream of living systems is denoted in what follows as the Thyroid Hormone Regulator or TH Regulator. Only models of this specific control system are considered here. There exist a fairly large number of published models of various other aspects of thyroid function, such as compartmental analyses of iodide metabolism and TH synthesis, distribution, and metabolism, but these are not within the scope of this work. In the various models reviewed in the following paragraphs, the symbols used to represent mathematical variables and paramaters have been changed from the original so that the different models can be more easily compared. In addition, it is assumed here that the reader is reasonably familiar with the general physiology of this system, which is described in the previous chapter of this book.

Several mathematical representations of the TH Regulator have previously appeared in the literature. All are parametric models, primarily concerned with the well known reciprocal interaction between the anterior pituitary and thyroid glands and the more recent of these models also include some of the currently postulated effects of the neuroendocrine organ, the hypothalamus, as an important organ of control and communication in this system.

The first published model is believed to be that of Danziger and Elmergreen in 1954 [3]. The author's purpose was to develop a mathematical theory of a mental disorder known as periodic relapsing catatonia. Some of the notable assumptions made in the development of this model were the following:

1. The system is homogeneous. (This simplifying assumption is implicit in the author's definitions).
2. In hypophysectomized animals the TH production rate is zero.
3. The hormones TH and TSH are lost or excreted at rates proportional to their concentrations.
4. TH and thyrotropin (TSH) inhibit and stimulate their target glands, the pituitary and thyroid, respectively, according to the Langmuir adsorption isotherm.
5. The pituitary secretes TSH at a constant rate, c, in the absence of TH inhibition.

JOSEPH J. DISTEFANO III AND EDWIN B. STEAR

The authors equate the rates of change of the levels of the hormones TH and TSH in the system to their production rates minus their loss rates and they obtain the following two simultaneous nonlinear differential equations for their model:

$$\frac{dx_1}{dt} = c - \frac{k_2 n x_2}{1 + n x_2} - \ell_1 x_1 \tag{10}$$

$$\frac{dx_2}{dt} = \frac{k_1 m x_2}{1 + m x_1} - \ell_2 x_2 \tag{11}$$

where

x_1 is the level of TH in the system at time $t \geq 0$

x_2 is the level of TSH in the system at time $t \geq 0$

ℓ_1 and ℓ_2 are the hormone loss constants; and k_1, k_2, c, m and n are positive, real constants.

Unfortunately, as the authors illustrate very elegantly, this model is inherently stable and consequently cannot exhibit the periodic oscillations believed to exist in the TH Regulators of catatonics. They do suggest, however, that the unknown source of instability in the TH Regulators of catatonic patients can be effectively removed from the system using a technique that they derive from their model. They propose that an amount of exogenous TH sufficient to shut off the secretion of TSH from the pituitary and, hence, shut off endogenous TH secretion from the thyroid be introduced into the system. In this manner the feedback loop between the two glands may be opened, thereby removing the ability of the system to oscillate.

Danziger and Elmergreen (1956) later published a second model of the TH Regulator [4]. They linearized the Langmuir adsorption terms in Equations (10) and (11) and added a third differential equation to represent the kinetics of an enzymatic mechanism by which they postulate that the pituitary stimulates thyroid secretion. With E chosen to represent the concentration of an activated enzyme, which they assume to be a peroxidase, and with a_1, b and k as positive real constants (and the other terms defined as before), they derive the following three differential equations to represent the model:

$$\frac{dx_1}{dt} = \begin{cases} c - a_1 x_2 - \ell_1 x_1 & \text{for } x_2 \leq c/a_1 \\ -\ell_1 x_1 & \text{for } x_2 \geq c/a_1 \end{cases} \tag{12}$$

$$\frac{dx_2}{dt} = bE - \ell_2 x_2 \tag{13}$$

$$\frac{dE}{dt} = mx_1 - kE \tag{14}$$

Equation (12) has two forms to account for the fact that the secretion rate of TSH from the pituitary must always be nonnegative. Thus, when $x_2 \geq c/a_1$, the pituitary secretion rate of TSH, $c - a_1 x_2$, is identically zero and the first form of Equation (12) degenerates to the second form.

The authors show, by deriving an appropriate set of relationships among the parameters, how these equations can have periodic oscillatory solutions of the relaxation type; and they again suggest, but in more detail, a technique based on their model for the treatment of periodic relapsing catatonia. They also associate certain pathological conditions such as hypo- and hyperthyroidism with variations in specific model parameters.

The model of S. Roston (1959) is presented as an example of a mathematical representation of endocrinological homeostasis [16]. It is homogeneous and is in general similar in structure and physiology to Danziger and Elmergreen's 1956 model [4], with three notable exceptions: it is linear second-order (no enzymatic reaction terms), it does not have periodic solutions, and it includes the possibility of autonomous secretion of both TSH from the pituitary and TH from the thyroid. In addition, Roston assumes that:

1.   TH bound to serum protein is part of the active pool of the hormone.

JOSEPH J. DISTEFANO III AND EDWIN B. STEAR

2. The physiological volumes V_1 and V_2 in which TSH and TH, respectively, are dissolved are constant over a short period of time.

3. The rate of secretion of TH is proportional to the rate at which TSH passes through the thyroid. This rate is therefore a function of both the amount of TSH in the blood and the rate of blood flow through the thyroid, which varies with sympathetic tone. However, for this model, the rate of blood flow is assumed essentially constant during a given short time interval.

4. The effect of the hypothalamus on the secretion of TSH from the pituitary can be expressed by changes in the value of a model parameter (a_1) which represents the sensitivity of the pituitary to TH inhibition. This is a mathematical statement of the so-called "filter hypothesis" of hypothalamic control over TSH secretion [1], which has been superceded by the "neurohumoral hypothesis" [9].

The equations of the Roston model are stated in terms of <u>amounts</u> of TSH and TH distributed homogeneously and instantaneously throughout the physiological volumes V_1 and V_2 they occupy and are given by

$$\frac{dx_1'}{dt} = f_1' - a_1'(x_2'/V_2 - x_{20}) - \ell_1'x_1'/V_1 \tag{15a}$$

$$\frac{dx_2'}{dt} = f_2' + a_2'x_1'/V_1 - \ell_2'x_2'/V_2 \tag{16a}$$

where x_1' is the amount (mass) of TSH outside the pituitary; x_2' is the amount (mass) of TH outside the thyroid; x_{20} is a physiologically standard value of TH (in concentration units); a_1' represents the sensitivity of the pituitary to TH inhibition; a_2' represents the sensitivity of the thyroid to TSH stimulation; f_1' is a constant secretion rate term, adjusting for autonomous TSH release from the pituitary when $x_2'/V_2 = x_{20}$; and f_2' is a constant secretion rate term, adjusting for autonomous TH release from the thyroid when $x_1' = 0$.

Equations (15a) and (16a) are easily written as hormone <u>concentration</u> equations (with unprimed symbols) by redefining the system parameters so as to absorb the volume symbols V_1 and V_2. This yields

$$\frac{dx_1}{dt} = f_1 - a_1(x_2 - x_{20}) - \ell_1 x_1 \tag{15b}$$

$$\frac{dx_2}{dt} = f_2 + a_2 x_1 - \ell_2 x_2 \tag{16b}$$

Roston indicates how these equations would be solved using Laplace transform techniques if the values of the parameters were known. He also points out that the model-system operates with a steady-state error in the level of TH; i.e., the steady-state value of x_2 obtained from the solution of Equations (15b) and (16b) is not equal to x_{20}, the assumed model-system "setpoint".

N. Rashevsky (1963) has presented a nonhomogeneous model of the TH Regulator in a discussion of a mathematical theory of the effects of cell structure and diffusion processes on the homeostasis and kinetics of the endocrine system [15]. He makes special reference to the influence of the endocrine system on periodic psychoses such as periodic relapsing catatonia. The author maintains all the basic assumptions of Danziger and Elmergreen (1956) and additionally introduces, with certain simplifications, the effects of the highly heterogeneous nature of the TH Regulator system. The chemical species reacting in this system are considered to be formed at different sites, having different physico-chemical properties, and these species are transported from site to site by the bloodstream. TSH is produced in N_p cells of the pituitary, which are surrounded by the intercellular fluid and the bloodstream, and a similar situation holds for N_t cells of the thyroid. The model incorporates certain permeability properties of the cells, diffusion properties within and surrounding the cells, and the size and shape of the cells.

The following simplifying assumptions are made in deriving the equations of the model:

1. The transport of components is effected only by free diffusion.
2. Transport dynamics through the intercellular fluid are neglected. (Prof. Rashevsky has recently successfully incorporated the intercellular fluid into his model [personal communication]).

174

JOSEPH J. DISTEFANO III AND EDWIN B. STEAR

3. The bloodstream has a constant volume, V.

4. The mechanism of action of TSH on TH production and TH on TSH production is purely catalytic. This means that the concentration of TH inside the cells of the pituitary, x_{2p}, is the same as in the blood, i.e., $x_{2p} = x_2$, and similarly $x_{1t} = x_1$ for the thyroid cells. If noncatalytic effects are assumed, the number of dependent variables in this model and therefore the number of equations and their resulting complexity are modified, but the general conclusions are the same.

The following four equations represent the model without the presence of the intermediate enzyme E introduced by Danziger and Elmergreen (1956) to allow for oscillitory solutions:

$$\frac{dx_1}{dt} = B\bar{x}_1 - Cx_1 \tag{17}$$

$$\frac{d\bar{x}_1}{dt} = \begin{cases} c - a_1 x_2 - A\bar{x}_1 + Jx_1 & \text{for } x_2 \leq c/a_1 \\ - A\bar{x}_1 + Jx_1 & \text{for } x_2 \geq c/a_1 \end{cases} \tag{18}$$

$$\frac{dx_2}{dt} = G\bar{x}_2 - Hx_2 \tag{19}$$

$$\frac{d\bar{x}_2}{dt} = a_2 x_1 - D\bar{x}_2 + Mx_2 \tag{20}$$

where $\bar{x}_1$ and $\bar{x}_2$ are the concentrations of TSH and TH in pituitary and thyroid cells, respectively; x_1 and x_2 are the corresponding concentrations of TSH and TH in the blood; and A, B, C, D, G, J, H, and M are constant parameters which are functions of the number, geometry, permeability and the diffusion properties of the cells of the pituitary and thyroid, the loss rate constants for TH and TSH metabolized in the tissues, and the volume V of the blood. The remaining parameters have previously been defined. This system of equations can exhibit sustained periodic oscillations for certain ranges of the parameters; and the introduction of the intermediate enzyme E is not necessary in so far as the existence of oscillations is concerned. Rashevsky also derives a system of six equations which include the production of the enzyme E as proposed by Danziger and Elmergreen (1956). For certain ranges of the parameters, this system also has undamped periodic solutions.

The author concludes from his equations that the size and shape of the cells of the glandular organs as well as their purely physical parameters such as permeabilities and diffusion coefficients must play an important role in the production of oscillations in the endocrine system. From this result, he suggests that variations of the geometry of the glandular cells or their physical properties, such as changes in their water content or the viscosity of the cytoplasm, may be the cause of periodicities in the system. Thus, an actual cure for diseases like periodic relapsing catatonia may be obtained if it is possible to restore normal conditions in the cellular environment of the allegedly diseased organs. This theory is potentially useful in that it possibly implicates certain factors such as drugs which affect the viscosity of cytoplasm or the membrane permeabilities, specific tumors, or purely mechanical trauma as being capable of permanently disturbing the homeostasis of the organism.

Norwich and Reiter (1965) have presented a second-order, piecewise-linear, homogeneous model, approximately equivalent to those already discussed, but with the parameters identified and assumptions stated somewhat more explicitly [14]. They define x_1 as the plasma concentration of TSH, in international units per liter, and x_2 as the plasma concentration of thyroxin (T_4), in micrograms of protein bound iodine (PBI) per 100 ml of plasma. All other parameters in the equations given below have been previously defined.

JOSEPH J. DISTEFANO III AND EDWIN B. STEAR

The authors make the following notable assumption, employing the neurohumoral hypothesis of hypothalamic control over pituitary TSH secretion: the pituitary autonomously releases TSH at a mass rate f_1V_1 which "is controlled by a supra-hypophysial center which is sensitive to the plasma concentration of thyroxin." They call this center a "thyrostat," they assume that it resides in the hypothalamus, and they assume that f_1V_1 remains constant over a short period of time.

The equations underlying this model are the same as (15b) and (16b), but with $f_2 = 0$ and $x_{20} = 0$. The authors mathematically transform these equations into a form in which it is easier to study variations of TSH and TH concentrations (x_1 and x_2) about their steady-state values ($x_{1\infty}$ and $x_{2\infty}$). They define

$$y_1 \equiv x_1 - x_{1\infty}$$

$$y_2 \equiv x_2 - x_{2\infty}$$

yielding the following (simpler) transformed equations:

$$\frac{dy_1}{dt} = - \ell_1 y_1 - a_1 y_2 \tag{21}$$

$$\frac{dy_2}{dt} = - a_2 y_1 - \ell_2 y_2 \tag{22}$$

Norwich and Reiter determine: the general solutions and characteristic equation of (21) and (22); the roots q_1 and q_2 of the characteristic equation, which on the basis of (unspecified) experimental work they assume are real; the responses to initial conditions (impulse responses) about $x_{1\infty}$ and $x_{2\infty}$; the extrema and times at which the extrema occur for these responses; and several relationships among the system parameters and the roots of the characteristic equation. On the basis of these derivations, the authors discuss the determination of the constant parameters of the model-system. They show how to estimate ℓ_2 from radioactive tracer experiments and indicate how the remaining parameters could be determined if both a reliable measure of TSH concentration were available and the roots q_1 and q_2 of the characteristic equation were known. They propose an experimental scheme to estimate these roots which is essentially equivalent to fitting transient experimental data to two exponentials.

In the most recent model of the TH Regulator, proposed by DiStefano (1966) and DiStefano and Stear (1968a),[5,6] it is assumed that the function of the system is to stabilize TH concentration in the plasma. This model incorporates the neuro-endocrine activities of the hypothalamus with regard to thyroid activity and pre-sumedly describes the dynamical characteristics of the passage of the hormones par-ticipating in TH Regulation between their glands of origin, their target organs, and the peripheral and portal plasma pools. The postulated neurohormonal secretion of the hypothalamus, denoted by neuroendocrindologists as Thyrotropin Releasing Factor (TRF), is included as a system dependent variable in addition to TH and TSH; and the additional possibility of humoral control over TRF secretion by detection of TSH and/or TH at hypothalamic sites is also considered.

The model is developed as a classical feedback control system consisting of a closed loop of components called the regulator and a lumped load on the regulator. The regulator consists of control elements, feedforward and feedback paths, and a directly controlled system. The control elements are the thyroid, anterior pitu-itary and hypothalamic organs; their intercommunicating channels - the peripheral plasma, hypophysial portal circulation and certain neurosecretory pathways within the hypothalamo-pituitary complex are the feedforward and feedback paths; and the directly controlled system is the TH content of the plasma pool. The lumped load on the regulator, called the indirectly controlled system, represents the physiolog-ical mechanism responsible for the net loss of hormones from the plasma to the pe-ripheral tissue space and the excretory pathways (see Figure 1).

The major assumptions used in formulating this model are as follows:

1. The pituitary, thyroid and hypothalamus function as hormone reservoirs and detectors. The hormonal control and feedback signals act only to alter the secretions rates from each organ.
2. TH secretion is stimulated by TSH and there is autonomous secretion of TH in the absence of TSH. TSH secretion is inhibited by TH, stimulated by TRF, and there may be autonomous secretion of TSH in the absence of TRF.
3. The hormones are lost from the plasma at rates depending on the physiolog-ical state of the tissues and other organs; these losses are interpreted as net loads on the regulator. Normal physiological-range load variations are small, slowly varying and may be assumed constant. Beyond the normal range of hormone concentrations, however, the loads are not constant but are nondecreasing functions of hormone concentration. This phenomenon of nonlinear hormone loss rates is interpreted as an adaptation (or self-adaptation) of the overall system to certain abnormal alterations in the

JOSEPH J. DISTEFANO III AND EDWIN B. STEAR

regulator components (e.g., partial thyroidectomy) because the quantitative character of the change is in a direction to maintain homeostasis.

4.   Circulatory feedback paths for TH and/or TSH acting at hypothalamic sites, thereby affecting TRF secretion, are possible.

5.   The hormones mix sufficiently rapidly and homogeneously in the plasma.

6.   Precursor materials for hormone biosynthesis (e.g., iodide ion) and hormone reserves are adequate for normal load variations; and biosynthesis of hormones is not a rate limiting factor in the normal system.

7.   The overall command input or setpoint for steady-state plasma TH concentration is variable in both the positive and negative directions. Changes in this setpoint may result from certain reflex activities and environmental variations believed to be initiated by various afferent inputs to the hypothalamus from the central nervous system (CNS); the mean value of CNS inputs is zero.

8.   The total level of TH binding proteins in the plasma is constant.

A schematic fluid flow diagram of this model is shown in Figure 2.

The symbols used in the mathematical model are defined as follows; all represent nonnegative quantities:

x_1 ≡ peripheral plasma TSH concentration.

x_2 ≡ peripheral plasma TH concentration.

x_3 ≡ portal plasma TRF concentration.

$\ell_1(x_1)$ ≡ coefficient of loss rate, or load, for hormone x_1 disappearing from the plasma, $i = 1,2,3$.

$a_1(x_2)$ ≡ a pituitary parameter representing the inhibitory effect of TH on the rate of pituitary TSH secretion.

$a_2(x_1)$ ≡ a thyroid parameter representing the stimulatory effect of TSH on the rate of thyroid TH secretion.

$p(x_3)$ ≡ the pituitary secretion rate of TSH due only to stimulation by TRF.

f_1 ≡ constant autonomous secretion rate of TSH from the pituitary into the plasma in the absence of TRF stimulation and TH inhibition of TSH secretion.

$f_2 \equiv$ constant autonomous secretion rate of TH from the thyroid into the plasma in the absence of TSH stimulation of TH secretion.

$e_1 \equiv$ rate of addition of exogenous TSH to the plasma.

$e_2 \equiv$ rate of addition of exogenous TH to the plasma.

The differential equations describing the dynamics of this TH Regulator model are:

$$\frac{dx_1}{dt} = e_1 + f_1 - a_1(x_2)x_2 - \ell_1(x_1)x_1 + p(x_3) \tag{23}$$

$$\frac{dx_2}{dt} = e_2 + f_2 + a_2(x_1)x_1 - \ell_2(x_2)x_2 \tag{24}$$

The terms e_1 and e_2 are normally zero in the physiological system. In addition to the physical realizability constraint that the hormone concentrations x_1, x_2, and x_3 are nonnegative, the net rate at which TSH is released into the plasma from all endogeneous sources must also be nonnegative:

$$f_1 + p(x_3) - a_1(x_2)x_2 \geq 0 \tag{25}$$

The nonlinear system defined by (23), (24) and (25) may be characterized as a feedback control system as shown by the block diagram in Figure 3. The broken lines represent the feedback paths to the hypothalamus which are still in doubt and the hypothalamus is simply denoted by a block because its effect on the overall system is represented in this model by its output x_3 or, more specifically, by $p(x_3)$, the pituitary secretion rate of TSH due only to TRF stimulation. The function $p(x_3)$ is dependent on x_1 and/or x_2 if the rate of TRF secretion is a function of the concentration of TSH and/or TH in the plasma.

Techniques for measuring and/or calculating the variables and parameters of the model described above are discussed or derived by DiStefano and Stear [6,7]. The quantities which are measurable by existing techniques are e_2, x_2, $\ell_1(x_1), \ell_2(x_2)$ and $a_2(x_1)$. The parameters f_2, and $a_1(x_2)$ in the steady-state, can be computed using the model equations; and e_1, x_1, f_1, and $p(x_3)$ in the steady-state, can be measured or calculated to within a single multiplicative constant, k. All calculations are in terms of quantities which are measurable under certain experimental conditions which are feasible and are defined or derived by the authors. The de-

JOSEPH J. DISTEFANO III AND EDWIN B. STEAR

rivations are designed to circumvent the difficulties in obtaining absolute values of the plasma TSH concentrations (x_1); only <u>ratios</u> of values of TSH concentrations are required and these can be reliably determined.

Perhaps the most important theoretical contribution resulting from the model is a proposal by the authors for two independent experiments to partially validate and further determine the structure of the TH Regulator [7]. The first experiment is designed to validate the steady-state form of the model equation representing pituitary-thyroid interaction. The experiment consists of determining the validity of the steady-state equation given below, which has been derived by the authors from model Equation (24). In this relationship [PBI] represents the steady-state plasma protein bound iodine concentration and [TSH] is the steady-state value for TSH concentration available from any assay for TSH. The subscript I represents a measurement in an intact animal, H in a hypophysectomized animal, and A in an animal subjected to an external stimulus capable of perturbing the steady-state TH and TSH levels. The latter condition may be obtained, for example, as a result of a constant exogenous infusion rate of TSH, or cold or electrical stimulation of the hypothalamus. The equation to be validated is:

$$\frac{[TSH]_A}{[TSH]_I} = \frac{\ell_{2A}[PBI]_A - \ell_{2H}[PBI]_H}{\ell_{2I}[PBI]_I - \ell_{2H}[PBI]_H} \tag{26}$$

Each of the quantities in Equation (26) is easily measured using existing techniques. If this equation cannot be validated, then the model represented by Equation (24) is incorrect. Such a result would imply that factors in addition to or other than the autonomous secretion of TH from the thyroid in the absence of TSH and stimulation of the rate of TH secretion from the thyroid by TSH are responsible for the normal steady-state level of TH in the circulation. These factors could include extrathyroidal sources of TH.

The second experiment is designed to determine the existence of possible humoral feedback paths from the thyroid gland to the hypothalamus and/or from the anterior pituitary to the hypothalamus; i.e., to show whether or not the mechanism responsible for TRF secretion from the hypothalamus is selectively sensitive to TSH and/or TH concentrations in the plasma (see Figure 3). If such feedback paths exist, their algebraic sign is also determined as a result of the experiment. The details of this experiment are lengthy and, consequently, only its theoretical basis is outlined here, along with a few pertinent equations.

The effect of the hypothalamus on TH Regulation is embodied in the term $p(x_3)$ in Equation (23); $p(x_3)$ represents the pituitary secretion rate of TSH due only to stimulation by TRF, x_3. Then, by definition, if the value of this function can be shown to be dependent on the value of x_1 or x_2, the rate of TRF secretion from the hypothalamus is dependent on x_1 or x_2. The experiment is designed to show whether or not $p(x_3) \equiv p$ is a function of x_1 or x_2.

Let p be written as $p(x_1, x_2)$ and consider the total differential Δp of p with respect to x_1 and x_2:

$$\Delta p \cong \left(\frac{\partial p}{\partial x_1}\right) \Delta x_1 + \left(\frac{\partial p}{\partial x_2}\right) \Delta x_2 \tag{27}$$

If p is a function of both x_1 and x_2, i.e., if both of the feedback paths in question exist, then a small differential change Δx_1 in x_1 and a small differential change Δx_2 in x_2 produces a differential change Δp in p that satisfies Equation (27) with $\partial p/\partial x_1 \neq 0$ and $\partial p/\partial x_2 \neq 0$. If $\partial p/\partial x_1 = 0$ and $\partial p/\partial x_2 \neq 0$, then only TH feedback exist; and if $\partial p/\partial x_1 \neq 0$ and $\partial p/\partial x_2 = 0$, then only TSH feedback exist. The algebraic sign of $\partial p/\partial x_1$ and/or $\partial p/\partial x_2$ is the sign of the feedback if $\Delta p \neq 0$.

An expression for Δp is derived from Equation (23) in terms of fourteen steady-state quantities, such as PBI levels, TSH levels and labeled hormone half-lifes, which are measureable under certain experimental conditions defined by the authors. The usual problem of obtaining absolute values for TSH concentrations is overcome by requiring the measurement of only ratios of TSH concentrations, as in the first experiment. Thus $\partial p/\partial x_1$ and $\partial p/\partial x_2$ are the only unknowns in Equation (27) and two independent experimental conditions are necessary to compute them. A sufficient pair of independent conditions can be experimentally obtained by introducing a small constant exogenous input rate, first of TSH (subscript α) and then of TH (subscript β), into the plasma of an experimental animal. In this manner, the steady-state TSH and TH levels may be perturbed. The differential quantities are defined by

$$\Delta x_{1\alpha} \equiv x_{1I} - x_{1\alpha} \tag{28}$$
$$i = 1,2$$

$$\Delta x_{1\beta} \equiv x_{1I} - x_{1\beta} \tag{29}$$

JOSEPH J. DISTEFANO III AND EDWIN B. STEAR

where the subscript I represents measurements made in the intact animal before the administration of exogenous hormone.

The overall experiment can be summarized in the following three steps:

1) Fourteen steady-state quantities must be measured under various experimental conditions.

2) Δp_α and Δp_β must be computed, using the measured values and the equations derived by the authors, and $\Delta x_{1\alpha}$ and $\Delta x_{1\beta}$, $i = 1,2$, must be computed from Equations (28) and (29). With these six values, $\partial p/\partial x_1$ and $\partial p/\partial x_2$ can be determined by solution of the following two simultaneous equations:

$$\Delta p_\alpha = \left(\frac{\partial p}{\partial x_1}\right)\Delta x_{1\alpha} + \left(\frac{\partial p}{\partial x_2}\right)\Delta x_{2\alpha} \qquad (30)$$

$$\Delta p_\beta = \left(\frac{\partial p}{\partial x_1}\right)\Delta x_{1\beta} + \left(\frac{\partial p}{\partial x_2}\right)\Delta x_{2\beta} \qquad (31)$$

3) Finally, the following six possible alternatives as results of the experiment must be considered statistically:

a) $\partial p/\partial x_1 = 0$ means there is no TSH feedback to the hypothalamus, i.e., $p \neq p(x_1)$.

b) $\partial p/\partial x_1 > 0$ means there is positive feedback of TSH to the hypothalamus.

c) $\partial p/\partial x_1 < 0$ means there is negative feedback of TSH to the hypothalamus.

d) $\partial p/\partial x_2 = 0$ means there is no TH feedback to the hypothalamus, i.e., $p \neq p(x_2)$.

e) $\partial p/\partial x_2 > 0$ means there is positive feedback of TH to the hypothalamus.

f) $\partial p/\partial x_2 < 0$ means there is negative feedback of TH to the hypothalamus.

INADEQUACIES OF THE MODELS AND SOME FURTHER SOPHISTICATIONS

The models of the TH Regulator summarized in the previous section certainly do not begin to describe nor is it their purpose to describe all of the physiology of this system. Also, as previously pointed out in this chapter and the previous one, many questions about the basic structure of this endocrine control system are still unanswered. However, several additional results reported in the biological literature can now be more or less easily incorporated into the DiStefano and Stear model as it is presently formulated [6].

It appears to be more in line with current thinking to consider the free fraction of TH rather than the total TH in the plasma as the controlled variable in this system. Thus, the stated purpose of the model-system should be to regulate the free TH in the plasma at a constant level. This additionally entails the incorporation into the model the dynamics of the process of the binding of TH to plasma proteins.

A further complication is that the model may be more useful, and more correct from the physiological point of view, if the two major components of TH, triiodothyronine (T_3) and thyroxin (T_4), are individually considered as controlled variables in this system; i.e., the system may dually regulate both T_3 and T_4 in a related but different manner. The evidence indicates that T_3 and T_4 are degraded at significantly different rates. Thus, their instantaneous ratio of concentrations in the plasma is not a constant.

The technique of model building for the TH Regulator, beginning with the most current model and incorporating one of the above modifications, is illustrated in the next several paragraphs.

In all previous mathematical models of the TH Regulator little or no consideration has been given to the binding of TH to specific plasma proteins. It is now known that many apparent anomalies of this feedback system can be explained in terms of the dynamics of the binding process [2]. For example, in human and primate pregnancy, PBI and hence bound TH levels are raised considerably, along with apparent but temporary thyroid hyperactivity. The TSH secretion rate, however, is not suppressed by this additional circulating TH and the free fraction of TH in the plasma remains essentially the same. This phenomenon is believed to be due to an increase in the level of TH binding proteins in the plasma, resulting in a significant increase in the proportion of bound to free hormone in the plasma. These findings and an increasing body of other evidence implicate the level of free rather than total or bound TH in the plasma as the negative feedback signal detected by the pituitary. Let the defined function of the TH Regulator, then, be to maintain the free fraction of TH in the blood at a constant level, while other mechanisms coupled to the TH Regulator, such as those regulating the level of hormone binding proteins, control the level of bound TH in the circulation. The mathematics of such a system is not difficult to derive, as is illustrated below, where a simplified model of the binding process is incorporated into the model first proposed by DiStefano and Stear [6]. The parameters $a_1(x_2)$, $a_2(x_1)$ and $\ell_1(x_1)$ defined for the previous model are also used in the new model and, for brevity, they are denoted by a_1, a_2 and ℓ_1, respectively.

JOSEPH J. DISTEFANO III AND EDWIN B. STEAR

For simplicity, no distinction is made between thyroxin (T_4) and triiodothyronine binding proteins, or between T_4 and T_3. Then B* represents the TH binding protein(s) species not bound to TH in the plasma and b* is its concentration. In addition, X_2 represents the bound and X_2^* the free TH species and x_2 and x_2^* their respective concentrations in the plasma. Note that since $x_2 \gg x_2^*$, then x_2 is approximately equal to the total TH in the plasma, $x_2 + x_2^*$. Thus the previous definition of x_2 as the total TH and the present one as the bound TH are for all practical purposes equivalent.

The stoichiometry of the simplified binding reaction is represented by

$$X_2^* + B^* \underset{k_2}{\overset{k_1}{\rightleftharpoons}} X_2 \tag{32}$$

where k_1 and k_2 are the reaction rate constants. To derive equations for the rates of change of x_2^*, x_2 and b* in the plasma it is convenient to consider each species as an individual compartment exchanging with several others, the overall system being an open one. Figure 4 illustrates the input, output and exchange vectors for these compartments and the differential conservation equations may be written by direct inspection of these flow diagrams.

Free TH is produced by the thyroid at a rate $f_2 + a_2 x_1$ and by dissociation of bound TH at a rate $k_2 x_2$; this second term is obtained by applying the mass action principle to the reaction Equation (32). Free TH is lost to the tissues at a rate $\ell_2^* x_2^*$, where $\ell_2^* \equiv \ell_2^*(x_2^*)$, and it is bound at a rate $k_1 x_2^* b^*$. Thus, the differential equation for free TH is

$$\frac{dx_2^*}{dt} = f_2 + a_2 x_1 + k_2 x_2 - \ell_2^* x_2^* - k_1 x_2^* b^*$$

$$= f_2 + a_2 x_1 + k_2 x_2 - (\ell_2^* + k_1 b^*) x_2^* \tag{33}$$

The differential equation for bound TH is obtained by direct application of the mass action principle to Equation (32) since the plasma is a closed system for bound TH; i.e., there is no input of bound TH from outside of the plasma and bound TH "leaves" the plasma only by dissociation to free TH. Therefore,

$$\frac{dx_2}{dt} = k_1 x_2^* b^* - k_2 x_2 \tag{34}$$

The rate of turnover of binding proteins in the plasma is, of course, dependent on the dynamics of the binding reaction, Equation (32). But there is an additional source or input of free binding proteins in the plasma. The increased concentration of estrogen in the circulation of pregnant women, for example, is believed to increase the concentration of binding protein in the plasma. The rate at which binding protein is introduced or produced in the plasma from all sources is denoted in this model by the function h. The loss rate of binding proteins is assumed to be zero as a first approximation because, although the proteins are metabolized, their rate of loss is relatively very small. From Figure 4 and Equation (32), the resulting equation for binding protein turnover is therefore given by

$$\frac{db^*}{dt} = h + k_2 x_2 - k_1 x_2^* b^* \tag{35}$$

The differential equation for TSH turnover in this new model is identical to Equation (23) of the old model, but with x_2 replaced by x_2^*. Thus, the new model is represented by the following four equations, plus the usual constraints of nonnegativeness of the concentrations of the chemical species and their production rates:

$$\frac{dx_1}{dt} = f_1 - a_1 x_2^* + p(x_3) - \ell_1 x_1 \tag{36}$$

$$\frac{dx_2^*}{dt} = f_2 + a_2 x_1 + k_2 x_2 - (\ell_2^* + k_1 b^*) x_2^* \tag{37}$$

$$\frac{dx_2}{dt} = k_1 x_2^* b^* - k_2 x_2 \tag{38}$$

$$\frac{db^*}{dt} = h + k_2 x_2 - k_1 x_2^* b^* \tag{39}$$

The steady-state solutions of these equations, writing ∞ subscripts for steady-state values and assuming $h_\infty \equiv 0$, are:

JOSEPH J. DISTEFANO III AND EDWIN B. STEAR

$$x_{1\infty} = \frac{\ell_{2\infty}^* [f_1 + p(x_{3\infty})] - a_{1\infty}f_2}{\ell_{1\infty}\ell_{2\infty}^* + a_{1\infty}a_{2\infty}} \qquad (40)$$

$$x_{2\infty}^* = \frac{\ell_{1\infty}f_2 + a_{2\infty}[f_1 + p(x_{3\infty})]}{\ell_{1\infty}\ell_{2\infty}^* + a_{1\infty}a_{2\infty}} \qquad (41)$$

$$x_{2\infty} = \frac{k_1 b_\infty^* x_{2\infty}^*}{k_2 + k_1 x_{2\infty}^*} \qquad (42)$$

Note that $x_{1\infty}$ and $x_{2\infty}^*$ are independent of b_∞^* and, in fact, these quantities are ex - actly equal to their corresponding values in the previous model. This means that the steady-state values of x_1 and x_2^* do not change as a result of a change in b_∞^*. Also, the last equation indicates that the steady-state bound TH concentration is directly proportional to the steady-state concentration of the binding proteins.

In summary, the equations derived above indicate that, to a first approximation, the TH Regulator responds to a change in the concentration of TH binding proteins by very rapidly modifying the concentration of bound TH after a brief, transient change in the free TH and therefore the TSH secretion rate. When the new equilibrium conditions have been established, the TSH and free TH concentrations are the same as before the change in binding protein levels. These phenomenon have been observed in pregnancy and in animals given estrogen.

REFERENCES

1.   Brown-Grant, K. (1957). "The Feedback Hypothesis of the Control of Thyroid Function." Ciba Found. Colloq. in Endocrin., 10, 97-116.

2.   Brown-Grant, K. (1957). "The Control of Thyroid Secretion." J. Clin Path., Suppl., 20, 327.

3.   Danziger, L. and G.L. Elmergreen (1954). "Mathematical Theory of Periodic Relapsing Catatonia." Bull. Math. Biophysics, 16, 15-21.

4.   Danziger, L. and G.L. Elmergreen (1956). "The Thyroid-Pituitary Homeostatic Mechanism." Bull. Math. Biophysics, 18, 1-13.

5.   DiStefano, J.J. (1966). A New Model of the Thyroid Hormone Regulator and a Proposal for its Experimental Validation. Ph.D. Dissertation, Dept. of Engineering, Univ. of Calif., Los Angeles.

6.   DiStefano, J.J. and E.B. Stear (1968a). "Neuroendocrine Control of Thyroid Secretion in Living Systems: A Feedback Control System Model." Bull. Math. Biophysics, 30, 3-26.

7.   DiStefano, J.J. and E.B. Stear (1968b). "On Experimental Determination of Hypothalamo-Hypophysial Control and Feedback Relationships with the Thyroid Gland." J. Theo. Biol., 19, 29-50.

8.   Goolden, A.W.G. (1954). "Radioactive Isotopes of Iodine and their Applications." The Thyroid Gland, R. Pitts-Rivers and W.R. Trotter, Eds., Butterworths, London, Ch. 15.

9.   Harris, G.W. (1964). "A Summary of Some Recent Research on Brain-Thyroid Relationships." Brain-Thyroid Relationships, M.P. Cameron and M. O'Connor, Eds., Little-Brown, Boston, pp. 3-16.

10.   Hsieh, H.C., (1965) "Synthesis of Adaptive Control Systems by Function Space Methods", Advances in Control Systems, Vol. 2, C.T. Leondes, Ed., Academic Press.

11.   Jacquez, J.A., Carnahan, D., and Abbrecht, P. (1967), "A Model of the Renal Cortex and Medulla", Mathematical Biosciences, 1, No. 2.

12.   Lee, E.S. (1968), Quasilinearization and Invariant Imbedding, Academic Press.

13.   McRuer, D.T., Graham, D., and Krendel, E.S. (1967), "Manual Control of Single Loop Systems: Part I", Journal of Franklin Institute, 283, No. 1.

14.   Norwich, K.H. and R. Reiter (1965). "Homeostatic Control of Thyroxin Concentration Expressed by a Set of Linear Differential Equations", Bull. Math. Biophysics, 27, 133-144.

15.   Rashevsky, N. (1963). "Mathematical Theory of the Effects of Cell Structure and Diffusion Processes on the Homeostasis and Kinetics of the Endocrine System with Special Reference to Some Periodic Psychoses", Nerve, Brain and Memory Models, N. Weiner and J.P. Schade, Eds., Elsevier, Amsterdam, pp. 244-256.

JOSEPH J. DISTEFANO III AND EDWIN B. STEAR

16. Roston, S. (1959). "Mathematical Representations of Some Endocrinological Systems." <u>Bull. Math. Biophysics</u>, <u>21</u>, 271-282.

17. Stark, L. (1969), "Pupillary Control System: Its Nonlinear Adaptive and Stochastic Engineering Design Characteristics," <u>Federation Proceedings</u>, <u>28</u>, 52-64.

18. Wilks, S.S. (1962), <u>Mathematical Statistics</u>, Wiley.

19. Yamamoto, W.S., and Raub, W.F. (1967) <u>Computers and Biomedical Research</u>, <u>1</u>, No. 1.

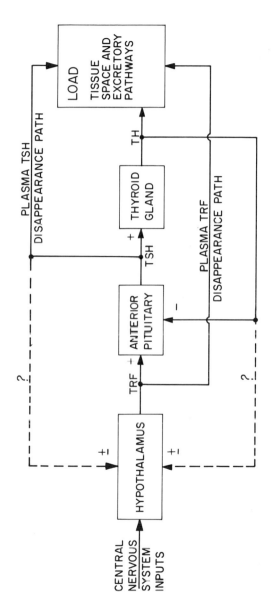

FIG. 1   Schematic Diagram of Thyroid Hormone Regulator

JOSEPH J. DISTEFANO III AND EDWIN B. STEAR

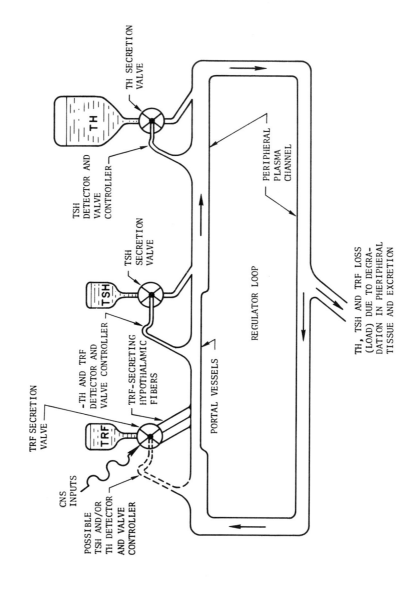

FIG. 2   Schematic Fluid Flow Diagram of Thyroid Hormone Regulator

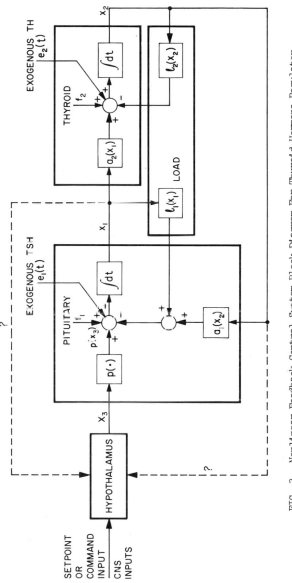

FIG. 3   Nonlinear Feedback Control System Block Diagram For Thyroid Hormone Regulator

JOSEPH J. DISTEFANO III AND EDWIN B. STEAR

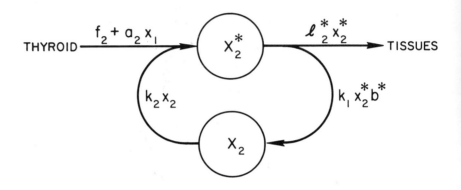

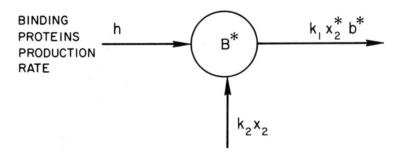

FIG. 4 Representation of Thyroid Protein Binding

S.M. McCANN, D.B. CRIGHTON,[1] S. WATANABE,[2] A.P.S. DHARIWAL, and J.T. WATSON
*Department of Physiology, University of Texas Southwestern Medical School
at Dallas, Texas*

7. REGULATION OF GONADOTROPHIN AND PROLACTIN SECRETION

INTRODUCTION

Our knowledge of the complex mechanisms which govern the secretion of the gonadotrophins is still in a relatively primitive state. This is in large measure due
to the absence of sufficiently precise, sensitive, and convenient methods of measuring blood levels of the gonadotrophins. It is difficult to study any regulation
unless what is being regulated can be measured easily and accurately. Yet, in spite
of these methodological limitations, we can now present a relatively clear outline
of the regulation of the gonadotrophins, as it has come from the combined efforts of
many investigators over a period of some thirty years. The following discussion will
first delineate some of the hormonal and environmental influences which can alter the
secretion of gonadotrophins, and will then present the evidence that these hormonal
and environmental influences act upon a hypothalamic regulatory area which modulates
the secretion of gonadotrophins.

It is necessary to deal with not one, but at least two, and perhaps three, hormones when discussing gonadotrophins. The follicle-stimulating hormone (FSH) promotes
the growth of the ovarian follicle beyond the stage of early antrum formation. By
itself, at least in the hypophysectomized rat, FSH evokes no hormonal secretion by
the ovary. A second gonadotrophin, the luteinizing hormone (LH), can act in the presence of some FSH to evoke further growth of follicles, ovulation, and formation of
the corpus luteum. LH stimulates the follicle to secrete estrogen, which rises to a

* Research in the authors' laboratory is supported by Grant AM 10073-02 from the
  National Institutes of Health and by a grant from the Ford Foundation and the
  Population Council.

1 Ford Foundation Fellow. Present address: University of Nottingham, Department
  of Agriculutre, School of Agriculture, Sutton, Bonington, Loughborough, England

2 Population Council Fellow. Present address: Cancer Center, Niigata Hospital,
  Dept. of Ob-Gyn, Kawagishicho, Niigata City, Japan.

S.M. McCANN, D.B. CRIGHTON, S. WATANABE, A.P.S. DHARIWAL, AND J.T. WATSON

peak just prior to ovulation. A third gonadotrophin, luteotrophin (LtH), is required
for the maintenance of functional corpora lutea and for the secretion of progesterone
in the rat and in other small rodents. In these species LtH appears to be identical
with prolactin. In women, convincing evidence for the identity of LtH with prolactin
is yet to be forthcoming. In fact, it has been shown that LH itself will increase
progesterone secretion by human corpora lutea in vitro. So, the question of the nature of LtH in man is still unsettled; however, for the purposes of this discussion,
the terms LtH and prolactin are used synonymously [43].

One of the primary goals of studying the regulation of the gonadotrophins is to
explain the fluctuating hormonal secretion during the mammalian estrous cycle or the
primate menstrual cycle. Although the following discussion will give a partial explanation for these cyclic changes, a complete explanation is still beyond our reach.
We shall consider all three of the gonadotrophins, i.e., FSH LH, and LtH; however,
since our knowledge of the regulation of LH is more complete than that for FSH and
LtH, we shall have much more to say about the first.

METHODOLOGY

Before proceeding further, it is perhaps worthwhile to say a little about the
various assays for gonadotrophins which are currently used. We are in the best po-
sition with respect to LH. Parlow [51] has developed a highly sensitive, specific,
and reasonably precise assay for LH: the ovarian ascorbic acid depletion technique.
This test is performed by injecting the solution to be assayed into immature, female
rats which have been pretreated with large doses of gonadotrophins.[3] The pretreatment is essential to enhance the ovarian sensitivity to the effect of LH. If the
material being tested contains LH, the ascorbic acid concentration in the ovaries
of the test animal decreases in proportion to the log-dose of LH injected.

The currently accepted assay for FSH is the ovarian weight method of Steelman
& Pohley [69]. Immature rats are treated concurrently with the FSH preparation to
be assayed and with a large dose of human chorionic gonadotrophin (HCG). This treatment with HCG augments the response to FSH and simultaneously blocks the response to
any LH which may contaminate the sample. In the presence of FSH, the ovarian weight
is increased. The method appears to be specific for FSH and reasonably precise, but
suffers from a low sensitivity, so that very large amounts of plasma are required to
obtain detectable levels of the hormone. Recently, in our laboratory, Igarashi [33]
has developed a mouse uterine weight method which is much more sensitive than the
Steelman-Pohley assay, but which is not completely specific for FSH. It does appear
to measure the FSH activity in plasma in which the quantities of LH present are too

low to interfere with the results obtained. In this method, HCG is also administered concurrently with the test sample to enhance the sensitivity to FSH and to block the response to LH, but the dose of HCG is much lower than that used in the Steelman-Pohley assay.

LtH must be assayed by either the systemic or local pigeon crop sac method. The sample is introduced intradermally over the crop in the local technique, and the area of the underlying crop gland which is stimulated is measured [25]. This method is sufficiently sensitive for assay for pituitary LtH, but is probably not sensitive enough to detect blood levels of this hormone.

Recently, new immunoassays have been developed which are applicable to measurement of gonadotrophins in body fluids and which will in all probability replace the bioassays. However, the methods described above have been used in most of the work to be discussed here.

FEEDBACK EFFECTS OF GONODAL STEROIDS ON THE SECRETION OF GONADOTROPHINS

In the intact animal, the secretion of FSH and LH by the adenohypophysis is held in abeyance by the feedback action of gonadal steroids. That such feedback effects are operative was perhaps first recognized by Moore & Price in 1932 [47]. In early work, alterations in the output of pituitary hormones in response to changes in the gonadal hormone titers was inferred from changes in the target gland size and structure. More recently is has been possible to examine gonadal steroid feedback by measuring the plasma levels of the gonadotrophins [41]. When the ovaries or testes are removed, both the plasma and pituitary levels of LH show a marked rise, the former from an undetectable level (Fig. 1). The plasma level is elevated within a week of gonadectomy, but appears to reach a plateau with no further rise over a period of months (Fig. 2). For unexplained reasons, the hypophyseal LH content continues to rise even after the plasma level has reached the plateau. Similarly, the plasma levels of FSH are markedly elevated in the castrated rat of either sex.

If one administers estradiol to the spayed female, beginning on the day of operation, the rise in plasma and pituitary LH can be prevented (Fig. 3); however, the quantity of estrogen required to accomplish this result appears to be slightly higher than that which is present physiologically, since it evokes vaginal estrus and a marked uterine enlargement (Fig. 3). This suggests that normally the inhibition caused by the estrogen is aided by another ovarian hormone which also plays a role in inhibiting LH. The logical candidate, of course, is progesterone. Progesterone alone has only a feeble inhibitory effect on LH release, and supraphysiological doses are required to lower plasma LH in the spayed rat. Pretreatment of an ovariectomized female with small doses of estrogen sensitizes the animal to the inhibitory effect of

S.M. McCANN, D.B. CRIGHTON, S. WATANABE, A.P.S. DHARIWAL, AND J.T. WATSON

progesterone; then under these conditions, doses of progesterone which appear to lie close to the physiological range have an inhibitory effect (Fig. 4). So we conclude that in the normal female the synthesis and release of LH are held in check by the combined actions of both estrogen and progesterone.

As might be predicted, the testicular androgen, testosterone, is capable of preventing the rise in plasma LH which follows castration in males. Here again, however, we have been puzzled by the observation that the dose required is greater than that required to return the weight of the sex accessories to normal. Possibly, small amounts of estrogen produced by the testes may synergize with testosterone in the normal animal.

The responses of castrates to administered gonadal steroids provide one of the pieces of physiological evidence for the belief that FSH and LH are in reality two discrete pituitary hormones and not merely artifacts provided to us by the biochemists. For example, Parlow [52] has shown that much larger doses of estrogen are required to lower pituitary FSH than to lower pituitary LH. Furthermore, the administration of testosterone, although lowering plasma FSH, produces a paradoxical elevation in pituitary FSH [6,23]. The explanation for these peculiar FSH responses is not yet at hand, and much more work must be done before a coherent picture of the effects of gonadal steroids on FSH secretion can be presented.

Still less is known about control of the secretion of LtH. For example, the effect of castration on the release of prolactin is unknown. One relevant fact which has been learned is that estrogen, given in rather high doses to intact rats, can elicit a state like pseudopregnancy. This is characterized by the presence of an enlarged pituitary gland, by enlarged functional corpora lutea, and by mammary development and secretion, which almost certainly indicate that the estrogen has evoked the secretion of LtH with its lactogenic action [18, 41]. Progesterone administration in normal female rats fails to cause reduction in size or other signs of involution of the corpora lutea, and has even been shown to evoke pseudopregnancy when administered in large doses. These findings have led Rothchild [64] to postulate that progesterone has a positive feedback effect on LtH secretion.

What happens when one combines treatment with estrogen and progesterone is apparently untested. In the normal animal, it is possible that the positive effects of gonadal steroids may enhance LtH secretion to aid in the maintenance of the corpora lutea during the last half of the estrous cycle. The problem then is that we know that gonadal hormones increase LtH release, but we know of nothing which inhibits it. Thus, the factors responsible for luteolysis at the end of the cycle are yet to be elucidated. It is interesting that hysterectomy leads to a prolongation of the life of the corpora in several species, and it has even been suggested that a luteolytic substance from the uterus may be responsible for terminating the life of the corpus luteum [1].

Another point which must be emphasized in any construction of hormonal relationships is that gonadotrophin secretion is cyclic in the normal human female and in many other mammals, such as the rat. Although plasma LH can not be measured during most of the estrous cycle in the rat, it rises to a readily measurable peak on the afternoon of proestrus [41]. The value obtained is as high as that found in ovariectomized animals. This cyclic burst of LH secretion which just precedes ovulation and is accompanied by a fall in pituitary LH (Fig. 5) has been attributed to a positive feedback of estrogen and progesterone operative at this stage of the cycle in the normal female. The estrogen and progesterone presumably arise from the maturing ovarian follicles.

Everett and his colleagues [18] have succeeded in advancing the time of ovulation in rats by the administration of either estrogen or progesterone. While the doses of estrogen which he used were much larger than the amounts present in the normal state of the animal, he achieved effects with relatively low doses of progesterone. Recently, we have observed an elevation of plasma LH within 6 hours of the subcutaneous injection of a small dose (1.5 mg) of progesterone administered during the preovulatory phase of the estrous cycle of the rat (Fig. 6). Ratner, in our laboratory (unpublished data, 1967), has been able to produce an elevation of plasma LH 24 hours after the subcutaneous injection of 1 μg of estradiol benzoate on the first day of diestrus.

Presumably then, the ovulatory surge of LH secretion may be caused by the stimulating effect of gonadal steroids. Why a positive feedback effect on LH secretion is seen under these conditions, whereas negative feedback has always been observed in the gonadectomized animal, is a mystery. Perhaps the rapidly rising titer of the steroids which occurs at this time is an important clue. We will return later to a further consideration of this phenomenon.

ENVIRONMENTAL FACTORS WHICH MODIFY GONADOTROPHIN SECRETION

Superimposed upon the influence of gonadal steroids on gonadotrophin secretion are the effects of environmental stimuli. Copulation induces ovulation in the rabbit, cat, and ferret presumably by a reflex activation of the hypothalamus. Another example of a neural influence on gonadotrophin secretion is the induction of pseudopregnancy in the rat following stimulation of the cervix or mating with a vasectomized male. Here a prolonged inhibition of FSH and LH secretion is coupled with enhanced LtH secretion. This provides one example of the frequently observed reciprocal effects of various stimuli on FSH, LH and LtH secretion.

S.M. McCANN, D.B. CRIGHTON, S. WATANABE, A.P.S. DHARIWAL, AND J.T. WATSON

Constant exposure to light, apparently acting via afferent fibers of the optic nerves, can abolish the estrous cycle in rats and induce a state of constant estrus. Actue and chronic stresses have also been reported to produce changes in gonadal and accessory organ weight which have been attributed to a reduction in the gonadotrophin output. We have been unable to find any effects of stress on LH secretion [59], but such effects may still occur although they may be limited to a reduction in FSH output.

Lactation, presumably put in operation via the stimulus of nursing, has a profound influence on gonadotrophin secretion. It is capable of lowering pituitary stores of both FSH and LH [53], and also of lowering the plasma levels of these trophins in the spayed female (these animals continue to lactate after ovariectomy) [40]. Since the gonadal steroids are absent in this situation, the effect is almost certainly a neurally mediated one. In contrast to its inhibitory effect on FSH and LH secretion, lactation clearly demands an augmented prolactin release. This is illustrated by the high requirements of the hypophysectomized, lactating animal for LtH [19] and by the acute drop in pituitary LtH content which occurs in intact rats following suckling [24]. This is another example of the reciprocal effects of various stimuli on the secretion of FSH and LH on the one hand and LtH on the other. Thus, a variety of factors influence gonadotrophin secretion in the normal animal and these are summarized in Table I. The possible negative feedback influence of gonadotrophins on their own secretion will be discussed later.

HYPOTHALAMIC CONTROL OF GONADOTROPHIN SECRETION

The observation that environmental changes could influence gonadotrophin secretion gave rise to the concept of central nervous control over the secretion of anterior pituitary hormones. More recently, the belief has grown that neural control of gonadotrophin release is not limited to the mediation of environmental influences, but also mediates the alterations in gonadotrophin secretion which occur during the menstrual or estrous cycle. Thus, opinions have swung away from the early conclusion that the pituitary is the master gland, and the view now prevails that it is itself under the control of the hypothalamus. Several lines of evidence substantiate this concept of hypothalamic control of gonadotrophin secretion.

First, electrical stimulation of the basal tuberal region will evoke ovulation in rabbits and rats [18]. This clearly indicates the existence of a pathway from the hypothalamus to the pituitary which can cause a release of gonadotrophins, but it does not prove that this is a normal pathway of hypophyseal activation.

Concrete evidence for the importance of the hypothalamus has come mainly from studies of the effects of hypothalamic lesions in man and lower forms--in particular, the rat. Hypothalamic lesions can induce precocious puberty in both man and rat, although there is considerable difference of opinion over the hypothalamic areas involved.

In adult rats, either of two syndromes can be produced [41]. Rostral lesions in the region just over the optic chiasm evoke vaginal changes typical of continual or constant estrus. In this situation, the animal appears poised on the brink of ovulation, but never goes beyond this point, and ovulation does not occur. The ovaries are filled with large follicles, while the estrous vaginal smear shows that these follicles are actively secreting estrogen. Apparently, in this situation the animal secretes relatively constant amounts of FSH and LH, which are responsible for follicular development and estrogen secretion, but the cyclic burst of LH secretion which produces ovulation is missing.

A much more profound interference with gonadotrophin secretion follows upon destruction of the basal tuberal hypothalamus. The key region here appears to be the median eminence (ME) of the tuber cinereum, the site of union of the hypothalamus and the pituitary stalk. If the ME is destroyed, the animal remains in a state of diestrus with a lack of follicular development. Apparently FSH and LH secretion have been turned off. This conclusion has been verified by placing lesions in the ME in ovariectomized rats. Two days after the placement of such lesions, the plasma FSH and LH are markedly lowered from the high levels induced by the ovariectomy. Also, if the operations are done in reverse order, the rise in plasma LH which normally follows ovariectomy fails to occur when animals with ME lesions are ovariectomized (Fig. 2).

Female rats with lesions in the ME show one change which stands in marked contrast to the atrophic condition of the ovarian follicles. It concerns the corpora lutea, which are large and appear to be functional. Proof of their function is provided by the fact that a deciduoma will form after uterine trauma. This decidual reaction can occur only when progesterone is present. It appears, therefore, that the animal with a ME lesion secretes LtH which stimulates progesterone secretion by the corpora. Moreover, there is evidence that this enhanced secretion of LtH stimulates the mammary glands; rats with these lesions do not show the mammary involution which normally occurs when a litter of infant rats is taken away from the mother [39]. Even in male rats, lesions of the ME will induce the secretion of milk [13]. This situation is clearly another example of the reciprocal effects on FSH and LH on the one hand, and LtH on the other. Apparently, when hypothalamic influences are removed by ME lesions, the secretion of FSH and LH is severely curtailed, whereas the secretion of LtH is enhanced (Fig. 7). Hypothalamic influences appear

S.M. McCANN, D.B. CRIGHTON, S. WATANABE, A.P.S. DHARIWAL, AND J.T. WATSON

to stimulate FSH and LH secretion in the normal animal while holding the secretion
of LtH in abeyance. This statement holds not only for the rat, but for the rabbit
[31] and human female as well [22].

HYPOTHALAMIC RELEASING FACTORS

One of the most striking recent advances in neuroendocrinology has been the
discovery that nerve cells of the hypothalamus secrete hormones which control the
secretion of the several trophic hormones of the pituitary gland. There is general
agreement among neuroanatomists that the anterior lobe has no secretory nerve supply;
but there is a means of communication between the hypothalamus and the anterior lobe.
It is via the hypophyseal portal veins, which provide a pathway for selective transmission of neurohumoral agents to the anterior pituitary. Although in the original
descriptions the blood was said to flow upward from the pituitary to the hypothalamus, in vivo observations of the direction of blood flow by Houssay, Biasotti and
Sammartino [32] in amphibia, and by Green & Harris [21] and by Worthington [74] in
mammals, have clearly established the direction as downward from the hypothalamus
to the pituitary. Since the vessels arise from capillaries in the ME and pituitary
stalk, substances secreted in this region clearly have preferential access to the
pituitary gland. More recently, additional vessels which arise from the neural lobe
proper have been shown also to perfuse the anterior lobe [11]. Consequently, Capillary blood from the entire neurohypophysis appears to pass to the anterior lobe.

LH-RELEASING FACTOR

When it was shown that either vasopressin (a hormone of the posterior lobe),
or a hypothalamic corticotrophin-releasing factor (CRF) extractable from the stalk-
ME (SME) region could trigger the release of ACTH from the anterior lobe, attention
was focused on the possibility that similar releasing factors might trigger the release of gonadotrophins (for review of literature see [27] and [42]. Such evidence
was soon forthcoming from two laboratories, our own and Harris's, which began work
on the problem independently at about the same time. We were able to show that the
same crude, acidic extracts of the rat SME which released ACTH were capable of de-
pleting ovarian ascorbic acid when injected into immature test rats prepared as for
the assay of LH [41]. A linear log-dose response curve was obtained (Fig. 8). Similarly prepared extracts from rat cerebral cortex had none of the activity found in
the hypothalamic extracts. Furthermore, the activity found in the hypothalamic extracts could not be accounted for by the presence of other physiologically active
substances such as epinephrine, Substance P, histamine, serotonin, or, in particular,
vasopressin or oxytocin.

The extracts of the SME region were shown to have no effect upon the ovarian ascorbic acid levels of hypophysectomized test rats. This, plus the observation that heating for 10 minutes in a boiling water bath inactivated rat LH while leaving unchanged the activity of the hypothalamic extract, clearly indicated that the material in question was not LH. At this point, the unknown active substance in the extract was termed the LH-releasing factor (LHRF).

In all the experiments performed up to this time, the extract had been injected directly into the immature test rats, which had been pretreated with large doses of gonadotrophins, and ovarian ascorbic acid depletion had been measured. Consequently, it was important to see if hypothalamic extracts could elevate plasma LH titers in other circumstances. In these experiments the extract was administered intravenously to adult rats, which were bled 10 minutes later. After centrifugation of the blood sample, the plasma was injected into the immature test rats to measure ovarian ascorbic acid depletion. The ascorbic acid depletion served as a measure of the plasma LH. An elevation in plasma LH occurred within 10 minutes of the intravenous injection of the extract into normal females, and it was also effective in ovariectomized rats in which the release of LH had been inhibited by lesions in the ME. This latter observation is an important one, because it indicates that the extract does not act via the nervous system, but presumably directly stimulates the pituitary.

No effect was obtained in similar experiments in which ovariectomized rats were used. We do not know the explanation for its ineffectiveness in this situation, but we hypothesize that the ovariectomized animal with its high level of LH secretion is already responding maximally to endogenously secreted LHRF and cannot respond further to the exogenously administered releasing factor. The factor failed to raise the plasma LH in hypophysectomized rats, another indication that it is not LH.

The quantity of LHRF in the hypothalamus is small. (This is, perhaps, not surprising, since the amounts needed are probably minute because the factor has preferential access to the pituitary via the portal vessels.) Consequently, the very sensitive ovarian ascorbic acid depletion assay is necessary to demonstrate activity after systemic injection of the hypothalamic extract. A different approach to this problem has been made in Harris's laboratory. They have implanted cannulae into the pituitary and injected minute amounts of hypothalamic extract into the gland. Campbell et al. [7], using rabbits, and Nikitovitch-Winer [50], using rats, were able to show that SME extracts would evoke ovulation in either species and that extracts from other brain areas were inactive. Vasopressin and oxytocin, as well as epinephrine, Substance P, histamine, and serotonin were inactive in their system (as in ours). Ovulation could not be induced by the systemic administration of SME extracts unless very large amounts were used. This rules out LH contamination of the extract as a factor in their results. These important experiments clearly point to

S.M. McCANN, D.B. CRIGHTON, S. WATANABE, A.P.S. DHARIWAL, AND J.T. WATSON

a hypophyseal site of action of the hypothalamic extract. The ovulation induced is presumably caused by LH; but since, as tested in hypophysectomized animals, ovulation is produced optimally by injections of mixtures of FSH and LH, it is apparent that their results can not be taken by themselves as proof of the release of LH alone. Release of FSH might have been responsible, at least in part.

An action of hypothalamic extracts in stimulating release of LH from pituitaries incubated in vitro has now been demonstrated in several laboratories [55,65] which adds further evidence for the view that the LHRF acts directly on the pituitary.

FSH-RELEASING FACTOR

Igarashi [34], in our laboratory, has made a systematic study of the possible FSH-releasing action of hypothalamic extracts. He has used prinicipally the mouse uterine weight augmentation method for estimating FSH, but has also confirmed his results with the ovarian weight augmentation method of Steelman and Pohley. An increase in plasma FSH was observed 10 minutes after the intravenous administration of SME extract. For the test animals he used ovariectomized rats in which the release of FSH had been inhibited, either by ME lesions or by the injection of large doses of estrogen and progesterone. Cerebral cortical extracts and the neurohypophyseal polypeptides, vasopressin and oxytocin, were inactive. Kuroshima, Ishida, Bowers & Schally [37] have confirmed these observations.

Mittler & Meites [45] and Schally's group [37], employing pituitaries incubated in vitro, have also found evidence for the FSH-releasing activity of hypothalamic extracts. So the FSH- and LH-releasing activity of SME extract has been demonstrated by both in vivo and in vitro tests.

Using these in vitro methods, the localization of the FSHRF and LHRF has been determined. FSHRF has been localized to the medial, basal, tuberal region, an area which contains the arcuate nucleus and ME [72] (Fig. 9). The neurosecretory cells which elaborate this factor may be located in the arcuate nucleus with axons which project to the ME. On the other hand, LH-releasing activity was localized to a broader basal zone which extended from the pituitary stalk forward to include the suprachiasmatic region (Crighton & McCann, unpublished data). Apparently the neurosecretory neurons which secrete the LHRF have a different distribution in the hypothalamus than those which secrete the FSHRF. They are distributed in the regions which if destroyed produce aberrations in LH secretion as already pointed out. Lesions in the suprachiasmatic region block the ovulatory discharge of LH and it may be that this area contains neurosecretory neurons whose axons project to the ME and release the LHRF which evokes ovulation. All of the neurosecretory neurons which con-

trol LH release can not be located here, since suprachiasmatic lesions do not block
LH secretion completely. In fact, the increase in plasma and pituitary LH which follows spaying occurs normally in rats with these lesions [2]. Consequently, we postulate that there are 2 sets of neurosecretory neurons which secrete LHRF. The first
set is localized in the suprachiasmatic region and is involved in the preovulatory
release of LH, the other located in the basal, tuberal region and is involved in the
basal release of LH and the altered release in response to the negative feedback of
gonadal steroids.

LtH RELEASE

Since the hypothalamus exerts an inhibitory influence over the secretion of LtH
or prolactin, one might expect to find a prolactin-inhibiting factor (PIF) in hypothalamic extracts. Pasteels in Belgium [54], and Talwalker, Ratner & Meites in this
country [70], have recently reported the discovery of PIF as follows: they found
that pituitaries incubated in vitro released large amounts of prolactin into the medium. This release of prolactin was inhibited by the addition of crude, acidic extracts of rat hypothalamus. Extracts of cerebral cortex were inactive, as were other
physiologically active substances found in the extract. In collaboration with
Grosvenor at the University of Tennessee, we have sought in vivo evidence for a PIF.
Grosvenor & Turner [24] observed that, in lactating rats, suckling for 30 min. induced an abrupt decrease in hypophyseal prolactin levels. We have observed that the
intraperitoneal injection of crude, acidic extracts of rat or beef hypothalamus into
lactating females 1-2 min. prior to the beginning of a suckling period can prevent
the suckling-induced decline in pituitary prolactin. Cerebral cortical extracts
were ineffective [26]. Consequently, it appears that, in addition to the LHRF and
FSHRF which stimulate gonadotrophin secretion, there is also a neurohumoral inhibitor
of prolactin release.

NATURE AND SIGNIFICANCE OF RELEASING FACTORS

To establish the physiological significance of the LHRF, it is desirable to
show that the quantity of the releasing factor stored in the ME fluctuates in situations associated with altered LH secretion. In our laboratory, Chowers [8] has
recently observed a lowering in the hypothalamic content of LHRF at proestrus, and
similar findings have been obtained independently by Ramirez & Sawyer [60]. Nallar
has even observed that plasma from long-term (more than six weeks) hypophysectomized
rats will deplete ovarian ascorbic acid in the immature rats of the Parlow test [48].
Plasma from recently hypophysectomized animals was without effect. If lesions were

S.M. McCANN, D.B. CRIGHTON, S. WATANABE, A.P.S. DHARIWAL, AND J.T. WATSON

placed in the ME of the long-term hypophysectomized animals, the plasma lost its capacity to deplete ovarian ascorbic acid. These results suggest that the hypothalamus
of the hypophysectomized rat in time secretes a large amount of LHRF. The secretion
is abolished by hypothalamic lesions. Thus, although much remains to be verified,
it seems highly likely that the LHRF is the physiological mediator for LH release.

If the pituitary is removed from its normal site and grafted to a location removed from the hypothalamus, gonadotrophin secretion is inhibited and prolactin secretion is enhanced as one would expect since the pathway for delivery of the releasing factors via the hypophseal portal vessels is no longer present. Recently, it has
been observed that multiple pituitary grafts at such a site in hypophysectomized rats
will maintain considerable gonadotrophin secretion as indicated by maintenance of
ovarian weight and the weight of sex accessory glands [20]. Does this means that the
pituitary has some residual gonadotrophic function in the absence of hypothalamic
control? We think not, since lesions in the ME of the hypophysectomized rat with
grafts leads to involution of testes and accessory organs (Beddow & McCann, unpublished data). Presumably, then, the residual gonadotrophin release by the grafts is
caused by gonadotrophin-releasing factors which reach the grafts via the systemic
circulation.

What is the chemical nature of the hypothalamic factors which affect gonadotrophin secretion? To try to answer this question, sheep and beef hypothalamii have
been used, since they provide larger quantities of the releasing factors than can be
obtained from rats. The LHRF is inactivated by the proteolytic enzymes, pepsin and
trypsin, which suggests that it may be a polypeptide. It is not inactivated by reduction with thioglycollate, a treatment which eliminates the biological activity
of the neurohypophyseal hormones, vasopressin and oxytocin, by splitting the di-
sulfide group joining the five-membered amino acid ring in their molecules. This
result again shows that the LHRF is distinct from vasopressin and oxytocin. The
technique of gel filtration through a column of Sephadex G-25 has been used in several laboratories to purify the LHRF. This procedure separates molecules primarily
according to their molecular size. When the adsorbed materials are eluted by wash-
ing the column, LHRF is eluted just prior to vasopressin, a result which suggest
that its molecular weight is slightly greater than that of vasopressin. Further
purification has been achieved by ion-exchange chromatography on carboxymethylcel-
lulose (CMC). The LHRF emerges from such columns as one increases the ionic strength
and pH of the eluting buffers. These results support the view that it is a basic
polypeptide [43].

The next question which should be answered is whether the factors, FSHRF and PIF, are identical with the LHRF. In our initial experiments employing gel filtration on small columns of Sephadex G-25, we were unable to separate the FSHRF from the LHRF. With the use of longer columns and different conditions of elution, Dhariwal et al. [14] have succeeded in separating the FSHRF from the LHRF. The FSHRF has been further purified by chromatography on CMC, a procedure which separates it from residual contaminating LHRF. Schally's group has obtained similar results and has prepared very highly purified FSHRF by application of several additional purification procedures [66].

It has proved to be more difficult to separate LHRF from PIF. The peak of both activities has resided in the same fraction after the gel filtration step, although there has been a tendency for the PIF to emerge from the column earlier. When the LHRF was chromatographed on CMC the tubes which contained LHRF were likewise active in inhibiting prolactin release [15]. Schally et al. [3] have claimed that a highly purified LHRF was devoid of PIF activity, but they have not reported the purification of this factor. It appears likely that the PIF will turn out to be a separate entity, but this question must be considered to be unresolved at this time.

The gonadotrophin-releasing factors and PIF are clearly separable from other hypothalamic factors which control the release of the other anterior lobe hormones.

One important question is whether or not these other hypothalamic neurohormones influence the response of the pituitary cells which secrete the gonadotrophins. We have begun to study this question by evaluating the effect of the other releasing factors on the basal and stimulated release of LH of pituitaries incubated in vitro. The addition of CRF, growth hormone (GH) - RF and growth hormone-inhibiting factor (GIF) failed to influence basal LH release or the LH released in response to LHRF. Preliminary experiments suggest that FSHRF likewise has no effect on the LH secreting cells (Crighton, Dhariwal & McCann, unpublished data). Consequently, it would appear that there is little if any interaction between the various releasing factors at the level of the pituitary cell. Further work is obviously needed to validate this generalization.

At least one primary action of the releasing factors is the stimulation of gonadotrophin release. An increased release can be measured in vivo within 5 minutes of injection of LHRF (Ramirez & McCann, unpublished data). Furthermore, LHRF is active in vitro in the presence of large doses of puromycin sufficient to block protein and LH synthesis (Crighton, Watanabe, Dhariwal & McCann, unpublished data). This clearly dissociates LH release from LH synthesis. The action of FSHRF is blocked by either puromycin or actinomycin [73], but it has been difficult to demonstrate a clear-cut effect of this factor on FSH synthesis, so that here again, a primary effect is prob-

S.M. McCANN, D.B. CRIGHTON, S. WATANABE, A.P.S. DHARIWAL, AND J.T. WATSON

ably on release.

The releasing factors do augment synthesis of pituitary hormones both in vitro and in vivo. For example, Evans & Nikitovitch-Winer [17] have obtained reactivation of pituitary grafts by infusion of hypothalamic extracts. Histological changes in the grafts were indicative of increased gonadotrophin storage in the face of increased release which must mean increased synthesis. It has not been determined if the effects on synthesis are secondary to increased release or are another primary action of the factors.

It appears highly likely that the hypothalamus exerts its control over hypophyseal secretion by secreting approrpiate releasing and inhibiting factors into the hypophyseal portal system to affect the secretion of each adenohypophyseal hormone. This method of control appears to extend to all the anterior lobe hormones.

SITE OF ACTION OF THE FEEDBACK OF GONADAL STEROIDS ON GONADOTROPHIN SECRETION

There are two obvious loci at which gonadal steroids might exert their feedback effects to inhibit the secretion of trophic hormones. Inhibition of either the hypophysis or the hypothalamic mechanism has been postulated. Several experimental approaches have been applied to the problem. The first of these is to implant minute amounts of steroid directly into the site under investigation. Rose & Nelson [63], the first to do this, reported a direct inhibitory effect of estrogen within the pituitary gland. Later List [38], and Sawyer and his colleagues [36], reported effects from placement of estrogen in the hypothalamus. They found little or no effect from the hypophyseal placements of gonadal steroids and concluded that the principal site of feedback was on the hypothalamus itself. Subsequently, Bogdanove [5] found that implants of estrogen directly into the anterior lobe would prevent a cellular change which occurs in the anterior lobe following removal of the ovaries. This change appears to be correlated with the hormonal changes already described. In agreement with Rose & Nelson, he concluded that the physiological site of the inhibitory effect of estrogen is located at the pituitary level, and argued that the effects obtained with hypothalamic placements of the steroid were caused by the absorption of the steroid into the portal vessels, which then distributed it to the pituitary gland, where the effect was actually exerted.

At about the same time, Ramirez & Abrams [58], in our laboratory, were able to show that implants of estrogen into either the ME region or into the pituitary gland would inhibit LH secretion and enhance the secretion of LtH. In ovariectomized rats with these estrogen implants, the plasma LH levels were lowered. In intact animals, LtH secretion was induced, as evidenced by the development of a pseudopregnancy syndrome characterized by persistent diestrus, enlarged corpora lutea, mucification of the vagina, and lobuloalveolar development and secretion in the mammary gland. We also noted that unilateral implants in the anterior lobe were associated with unilateral enlargement of the gland which at face value would appear to be clear evidence of a local effect. Kanematsu & Sawyer [36], working with ovariectomized rabbits, also found that hypothalamic implants of estrogen lowered plasma LH levels. On the other hand, they found increased storage without enhanced release of LtH in intact animals with hypothalamic implants of estrogen, whereas pituitary placements of the steroid caused LtH release accompanied by low hypophyseal content [35]. The cause of this difference in behavior of LtH in the two species remains obscure. Meites and his associates [49] have found that estrogen applied to rat pituitaries incubated in vitro will augment LtH release, which agrees with our in vivo findings. I believe that it is safe to conclude from this discussion that estrogen can act directly at the pituitary level. Whether there is also an action at the hypothalamic level cannot be decided conclusively from these data, in view of possible absorption into the portal vessels with an action on the pituitary.

Other lines of evidence, however, have recently led to the conclusion that these steroids must also act at a site other than the pituitary gland, presumably on the hypothalamus. If the inhibition were exerted only at the pituitary level, one would expect that treatment of ovariectomized rats with large doses of gonadal steroids would block the response to LHRF or FSHRF given by injection. This is not the case. Varying doses of estrogen, which lowered the plasma LH and FSH in these ovariectomized rats, were incapable of preventing the elevation of plasma LH and FSH that followed intravenous administration of LHRF or FSHRF. Even when progesterone (25 mg) was administered along with estradiol benzoate (50 µg), the LHRF or FSHRF was still effective. In fact, the ovariectomized, estrogen-progesterone-blocked rat is supersensitive to the action of LHRF. Such animals respond to the extract made from as little as 0.015 of 1 rat SME by showing LH release, whereas injection of 0.4 of 1 SME is required for LH secretion in the immature rats which are routinely used for this test [34,41].

Furthermore, the sensitivity of the pituitary to the LHRF appears to be reasonably constant throughout the estrous cycle [2]. Consequently, it would seem that the enhanced release of LH prior to ovulation is caused by an increased release of LHRF from the positive feedback of gonadal steroids rather than by a constant release of LHRF and an increased pituitary sensitivity induced by steroids at the time of the preovulatory discharge of LH.

S.M. McCANN, D.B. CRIGHTON, S. WATANABE, A.P.S. DHARIWAL, AND J.T. WATSON

In other studies it has been observed that implants of estradiol or testosterone into the ME can lower the content of LHRF stored in the ME. A similar effect was obtained with large doses of systemically administered testosterone [8]. Effects of castration and administration of steroids on the content of FSHRF in the hypothalamus have also been reported [46]. A fall in the content of stored LHRF has been observed at proestrus which is consistent with a discharge of the factor to induce LH release and ovulation [8,60].

It does appear likely, then, that there are two sites of action of gonadal steroids on gonadotrophin secretion, and that the effects are mediated both at the hypothalamic and hypophyseal levels. As a working hypothesis we assume that the hypothalamic site is the more sensitive and is the one involved in mediating the physiological effects of these steroids.

There is good evidence for the view that the negative feedback effects of these steroids on gonadotrophin release are mediated predominantly in the basal tuberal region. Most of these evidence has already been cited and is summarized in Table II. It is noteworthy that gonadotrophin secretion continued but ovulation was blocked when the basal tuberal region was isolated from the rest of the brain by means of an ingenious knife (developed by Halasz). Increased LH release follows castration in this preparation, just as in normal rats [28]. This indicates by a still different approach that the negative feedback is localized to either the basal tuberal region itself or the pituitary gland.

The localization of the positive feedback effect of gonadal steroids on LH secretion is less certain, although we believe it is probably exerted in the suprachiasmatic region. The evidence is summarized in Table III, and much of it has already been documented. In addition to the capacity of lesions in this area to block ovulation, and of stimulation here to evoke it, it has now been shown that a knife cut which separates the suprachiasmatic region from the basal tuberal hypothalamus will block ovulation [28]. The most direct evidence is that estrogen implants into this area can evoke precocious puberty [68], which is known to be accomplished by increased gonadotrophin discharge.

POSSIBLE NEGATIVE FEEDBACK OF GONADOTROPHINS AND PROLACTIN TO INHIBIT THE PITUITARY

As in the case of most other pituitary hormones, evidence is accumulating to indicate that LH may feedback negatively to inhibit its own secretion. In order to be meaningful, such experiments must be carried out in castrates to eliminate effects of gonadal steroids secreted secondarily as the result of LH. The results of two studies have been published [9,12] in which a rather modest fall in pituitary LH was demonstrated. In one [12] plasma LH was reported to be lowered in a single experiment, whereas in the other study no effect on plasma LH was observed [9]. In our own work on this problem (McCann et al., unpublished data), a small decline in pituitary LH was observed which was of borderline significance. No consistent significant effect of these hypothalamic implants of LH on plasma LH was observed in 12 separate experiments. Large doses of LH were also administered intravenously to ovariectomized and hypophysectomized rats and assays were performed after sufficient time had elapsed to allow for disappearance of the exogenous LH. A borderline lowering of plasma LH was observed in nine experiments, and the circulating LHRF found in plasma of the chronically hypophysectomized rats disappeared. Ramirez et al. [62] have just reported that LH injections can alter hypothalamic unit activity in the basal tuberal region, an observation which suggests a feedback action on this portion of the brain.

Taken altogether, the data indicate that this autofeedback of LH does exist, but since the observed effects were small, it would appear to be inoperative except at levels of LH secretion at the upper limit of the physiological range. Perhaps this is one factor which causes plasma LH to plateau at a high level in the chronically ovariectomized rat and which serves to shut off LH secretion at the end of the ovulatory burst. From a functional standpoint it seems self-defeating for such a feedback to be operative at lower plasma levels of hormone necessary for it to exercise its effect on the target organs. Whether or not this feedback operates via sensing in the hypothalamus of peripheral circulating levels of LH or via delivery of high levels of LH to the hypothalamus either by retrograde flow in portal vessels or by diffusion from the pars tuberalis remains to be seen.

As in the case of LH, FSH may act on the hypothalamus to inhibit its own secretion, for Corbin & Story [10] have reported declines in hypothalamic FSHRF and pituitary FSH in intact rats with implants of FSH into the ME. Control implants were ineffective. Transplantable pituitary tumors which secrete excessive prolactin likewise depress prolactin levels in the host's pituitary [44].

SEXUAL DIFFERENTION OF THE HYPOTHALAMUS

Although a cyclic release of LH appears to induce ovulation periodically in spontaneously ovulating females of such species as man and the rat, it is generally believed that the secretion of gonadotrophin by males is relatively constant. This can be shown by grafting ovaries into a castrated male: although the ovaries become filled with large follicles, ovulation fails to occur. If vaginal epithelium has also been grafted into such a male, it will be observed to show persistent cornification. By contrast, similar ovarian and vaginal grafts in spayed females show evi-

S.M. McCANN, D.B. CRIGHTON, S. WATANABE, A.P.S. DHARIWAL, AND J.T. WATSON

dence of cyclic activity. What is the reason for this basic difference in the behavior of the gonadotrophin-regulating mechanism in males and females? Pfeiffer, in
the mid-1930's [56], gained the first insight into the mechanism when he found, using
male rats castrated at birth, that ovarian grafts would later show evidence of cyclic
behavior. Conversely, if testes were transplanted into females at birth, the females
bearing both their own ovaries and engrafted testes failed to show ovarian cycles when
adult, and instead showed constant vaginal estrus and follicles without corpora lutea
in their ovaries. On the other hand, if females wer ovariectomized at birth, ovaries
grafted into them when they had reached adulthood gave evidence of cyclic behavior.

These findings have been confirmed and extended by later workers, in particular
by Yazaki, by Gorski, and by Harris & Levine [30]. They suggest that an intrinsic
cyclic mechanism is inherent in females, but that male hormone from the testis can
convert this to the male, acyclic pattern. Barraclough [4] and others have indeed
shown that injection of a single minute dose of testosterone into newborn females
during the first few days of life is sufficient to block cyclic gonadotrophin secretion, so that the adults show persistent vaginal estrus and the presence of only follicles in the ovary. Since later injections of an androgen fail to evoke this syndrome, the concept has developed that there is a critical period during the first few
days of life, in which androgen can induce the acyclic pattern of gonadotrophin secretion.

One might argue that the defect in these so-called androgenized females is located in the ovary or in the hypophysis; however, this argument is refuted, since
grafting of either the ovary or the pituitary of such an androgenized female into a
normal recipient combined with removal of its own corresponding gland is followed by
a return to normal function of the graft in question. By exclusion, the most likely
locus for the defect in the androgenized female, therefore, is in the hypothalamus.
It will be remembered that lesions in the suprachiasmatic region evoke a similar state
characterized by persistent vaginal estrus. Barraclough has shown that electrical
stimulation of this same suprachiasmatic region fails to evoke ovulation in these
androgenized female rats, although it readily does so in normal females. The androgenized rat, however, can be made to ovulate by electrical stimulation of the
basal tuberal region, so apparently only the rostral region is refractory to such
stimulation. Barraclough & Gorski postulate that neonatal androgen from the infantile testis alters the nature of this suprachiasmatic region, so that the cyclic
feminine pattern of gonadotrophin secretion is changed to the male acyclic pattern.
Thus, in addition to feeding back on the hypothalamus to inhibit gonadotrophin secretion, androgens appear to have an inductive influence on the infantile hypothalamus which can alter its subsequent pattern of behavior. Wagner, Erwin & Critchlow

[71] have provided additional evidence for this point of view. They demonstrated that testosterone implants in the suprachiasmatic region of newborn females could pro-duce' the syndrome.

MECHANISM OF PUBERTY

One of the baffling problems in studies of the control of the endocrinology of reproduction has been the mechanism by which puberty is induced. What prevents pre-mature secretion of gonadotrophin and resultant precocious puberty at a time when the organism is ill equipped for assuming reproductive functions? Now that we have examined the mechanisms which regulate gonadotrophin secretion, we can approach this mystery.

Certain facts appear to be well established. First, gonadotrophin excretion is low in infancy and rises at puberty. Yet the immature gonad (at least after a very early unresponsive period) is quite capable of responding to gonadotrophins and of developing to maturity. Moreover, the immature hypophysis is similarly capable of premature secretion of gonadotrophins, for when Harris & Jacobsohn [29] hypophysec-tomized female rats and placed the pituitaries of their infant offspring in the sella turcica, the adult females again began to show estrous cycles after only a short de-lay. Finally, hypothalamic lesions in the infantile human of either sex or in in-fantile rats have been shown to evoke precocious puberty. These facts indicate that the immature gonad and pituitary are capable of assuming adult levels of function. Presumably, during the prepuberal period, the pituitary is not being stimulated by the hypothalamus [16].

Ramirez [57] has studied this problem in our laboratory in regard to LH secre-tion. First, he found that castration of both male and female infantile rats at the tenth postpartum day was followed within two weeks by elevated levels of plasma LH which were as high as those found in adult castrates (Fig. 10). This occurred at an age (24 days) when an intact animal would still be sexually infantile. Apparently castration removed a brake on gonadotrophin secretion in these immature animals. Castration was also followed by a definite, though small, reduction in weight of the infantile accessory sex organs, which indicated that the infantile gonads must have been secreting small amounts of gonadal steroids.

LH was present in the pituitary and LHRF in the hypothalami of the immature rats which had not been castrated, so we concluded that all LH-releasing machinery was present in the immature rat, but that something was holding the secretion of gonado-trophins in check.

S.M. McCANN, D.B. CRIGHTON, S. WATANABE, A.P.S. DHARIWAL, AND J.T. WATSON

Ramirez then compared the sensitivity of adult and immature castrates to the inhibitory action of gonadal steroids on LH secretion, and found that the sensitivity to estradiol was two to three times greater in the immature females than in the adults. For testosterone in males, the difference in sensitivity was three-to fourfold (Fig. 10). In these experiments the dosage of hormonal replacement therapy was expressed in terms of body weight to correct for the great disparity in weight between the adult and the immature animals.

These experimental results can be explained by postulating that at puberty the hypothalamus becomes less sensitive to the negative feedback by gonadal steroids. At this time the low levels of steroid secreted by the immature gonad are no longer adequate to hold the gonadotrophin secretion in check. Augmented gonadotrophin secretion follows, which is stabilized at the adult level when the gonadal steroid titers reach the higher adult value, which is once again capable of inhibiting further gonadotrophin release. This hypothesis implies that a change in the hypothalamic sensitivity to gonadal steroids is a major factor in the development of puberty. Unfortunately, we are unable to measure in blood the levels of gonadal steroids which are actually produced by these injections, and this constitutes a possible loophole in the foregoing argument. The results could be explained equally well by postulating an altered metabolism of gonadal steroids at puberty. If the rate of degradation of gonadal steroids were increased at puberty, an apparent decrease in sensitivity to the feedback action of the steroids would also be seen.

In an important study Smith & Davidson [67] have just shown with implanation of gonadal steroids into the hypothalamus that smaller quantities will inhibit gonadotrophin secretion in immature animals than in adults. Consequently, it appears that the reset hypothesis is correct.

Even if the reset hypothesis is correct, it still leaves us completely ignorant of the factors which bring about this altered hypothalamic sensitivity at puberty. That the gonadal steroids themselves may induce the lowered sensitivity which occurs at puberty is suggested by some recent experiments of Ramirez & Sawyer [61] who have observed that minute doses of estrogen administered to infantile female rats will advance puberty.

CONCLUDING REMARKS

It can be seen from the preceding discussion that a complex interplay of humoral and neural factors influences the hypothalamic mechanism which governs the secretion of hypophyseal gonadotrophins. However, this complex interplay in a three-tiered hierarchy of endocrinological control begins to reveal the complexity necessary to account for the varieties of temporal organization in the sexual functions. The system must account for the acyclic pattern characteristic of males, the various forms of periodic female cycles, the problems of the appearance of puberty, and in the end, the acyclic pattern of the senescent female. The tale is still fragmentary, but these fragments reveal that the hypothalamus plays the important role. Beginning in the neonatal period, androgen from the infantile testis may act upon the rostral hypothalamus to convert a female, cyclic hypothalamic pattern into a male, acyclic one. As the animal matures, a declining hypothalamic sensitivity to the negative feedback action of gonadal steroids may set the stage for the augmented gonadotrophin secretion that initiates puberty. In the adult animal, there is a negative feedback of gonadal steroids on the release of FSH and LH. Under some circumstances, however, a positive feedback of estrogen and progesterone on LH secretion can also be demonstrated; it is thought to evoke the ovulatory burst of LH secretion at mid-cycle. Both estrogen and progesterone appear to have mainly a stimulatory or positive feedback action on LtH secretion. In most of the circumstances thus far analyzed, there is a reciprocal relationship between the secretion of FSH and LH on the one hand and LtH on the other. This appears to be a consequence of the fact that both hormonal and environmental influences act upon a hypothalamic mechanism, so as to stimulate secretion of FSH and LH, and to inhibit secretion of LtH, or vice versa. The hypothalamic control over secretion is mediated by means of neurohumoral agents FSHRF, LHRF and PIF, which upon secretion into the hypophyseal portal vessels, are responsible for the observed alterations in output of gonadotrophins from the adenohypophysis.

The entire system for regulation of LH secretion is illustrated in a physiologist's type of diagram (Fig. 11). This diagram omits the regulation for FSH, which is quite similar to that for LH, and also does not consider the situation with respect to prolactin (LtH) which is more or less the opposite of the regulation of FSH and LH.

If one utilizes an engineering type of diagram (Fig. 12), the entire picture for all three hormones can be conveniently depicted. The concept of a lumped parameter physical system is shown by a signal flow diagram or network whose branches represent the physical elements. The network contains the physical elements defined by constant or variable parameters that can be represented by a finite number of degrees of freedom.

The block diagram provides a pictorial relationship between the cause-and-effect relationship between the input and output of the system. The arrows indicate an implied unilateral property to the system component involved.

From such diagrams are eventually derived the integro-differential equations of motion of the system. The possible cross-talk between these three feedforward channels has not been included because of the lack of clear physiological evidence for

S.M. McCANN, D.B. CRIGHTON, S. WATANABE, A.P.S. DHARIWAL, AND J.T. WATSON

this interaction.

TABLE I

REGULATION OF LH SECRETION IN THE NORMAL RAT OR HUMAN

1) Relatively constant secretion in the male
2) Cyclic discharge of LH in the female with a peak discharge just prior to ovulation (which is caused by the preovulatory discharge)
3) Cyclic discharge probably caused by stimulatory (positive feedback) of estrogen and progesterone during the preovulatory phase of the estrous (menstrual) cycle
4) There is an inhibitory or negative feedback action of gonadal steroids since castration leads to enhanced release and synthesis of LH, whereas gonadal steroids can inhibit this release
5) There may be a negative feedback of LH on its own secretion operative at high levels of LH release as for example at ovulation and in the castrate
6) Gonadotrophin secretion is low in prepuberal animals and its rise to adult levels initiates puberty
7) Environmental factors such as light and nursing influence gonadotrophin secretion

TABLE II

EVIDENCE THAT THE BASAL TUBERAL REGION IS THE PRINCIPAL SITE OF THE INHIBITORY ACTION OF GONADAL STEROIDS ON LH SECRETION

1) Stimulation of this area gives LH secretion
2) Lesions in this area block LH secretion and prevent the response to castration
3) Implants of gonadal steroids into this region inhibit LH release and synthesis and are associated with a decrease in LH-RF stored in the stalk-median eminence
4) Implants of steroids in the preoptic region fail to inhibit LH secretion
5) Lesions of the preoptic or anterior hypothalamic region fail to block the increased LH secretion as a result of castration
6) The isolated basal tuberal region is capable of increasing LH secretion as a result of castration

TABLE III

EVIDENCE THAT THE PREOPTIC REGION IS THE SITE OF THE STIMULATORY ACTION OF GONADAL
STEROIDS ON LH SECRETION

1) Stimulation of this region causes ovulation

2) Lesions in this area block ovulation

3) Isolation of this area by deafferentation of the basal tuberal region blocks
ovulation

4) Estrogen implants in this area can evoke precocious puberty

REFERENCES

1. Anderson, L.L., A.M. Bowerman and R.M. Melampy. Neuroutero-ovarian relationships. IN: Advances in Neuroendocrinology, 345-373, Nalbandov, A.V., (ed).
University of Illinois Press: Urbana, 1963.

2. Antunes-Rodrigues, J., A.P.S. Dhariwal and S.M. McCann. Effect of purified
luteinizing hormone-releasing factor (LH-RF) on plasma LH activity at various
stages of the estrous cycle of the rat. Proc. Soc. Exp. Biol. Med. 122:1001-
1004, 1966.

3. Arimura, A., T. Saito, E.E. Müller, C.Y. Bowers, S. Sawano and A.V. Schally.
Absence of prolactin-release inhibiting activity in highly purified LH-releasing
factor. Endocrinology 80: 972-974, 1967.

4. Barraclough, C.A., Modifications in the CNS regulation of reproduction after
exposure of prepubertal rats to steroid hormones. Rec. Prog. Hor. Res. 22:503-
539, 1966.

5. Bogdanove, E.M., Direct gonad-pituitary feedback: an analysis of effects of in-
tracranial estrogenic depots on gonadotroph secretion. Endocrinology 73:696-712,
1963.

6. Ramirez, V.D. and C.H. Sawyer., Changes in hypothalamic luteinizing hormone releasing factor (LHRF) in the female rat during puberty. Endocrinology 78:958-
964, 1966.

7. Campbell, H.J., G. Feuer and G.W. Harris., The effect of intrapituitary infusion
of median eminence and other brain extracts on anterior pituitary gonadotrophic
secretion. J. Physiol. (London) 170

8. Chowers, I. and S.M. McCann. Content of luteinizing hormone-releasing factor
and luteinizing hormone during the estrous cycle and after changes in gonadal
steroid titers. Endocrinology 76:700-708, 1965.

9. Corbin, A., Pituitary and plasma LH of ovariectomized rats with median eminence
implants of LH. Endocrinology 78:983-896, 1966.

10. Corbin, A., and J.C. Story. "Internal" feedback mechanism: response of pituitary FSH and of stalk-median eminence follicle stimulating hormone-releasing
factor to median eminence implants of FSH. Endocrinology 80:1006-1012, 1967.

S.M. McCANN, D.B. CRIGHTON, S. WATANABE, A.P.S. DHARIWAL, AND J.T. WATSON

11. Daniel, P.M. and M.M.L. Prichard. Anterior pituitary necrosis. Infarction of the pars distalis produced experimentally in the rat. Quart. J. Exptl. Physiol. 41:215-229, 1956.

12. David, M.A., F. Fraschini and L. Martini. Control of LH secretion: role of a "short" feedback mechanism. Endocrinology 78:55-60, 1966.

13. deVoe, W.F., V.D. Ramirez and S.M. McCann. Induction of mammary secretion by hypothalamic lesions in male rats. Endocrinology 78:158-164, 1965.

14. Dhariwal, A.P.S., R. Nallar, M. Batt and S.M. McCann. Separation of follicle stimulating hormone-releasing factor from luteinizing hormone-releasing factor. Endocrinology 76:290-294, 1965.

15. Dhariwal, A.P.S., C. Grosvenor, J. Antunes-Rodriques and S.M. McCann. Purification of ovine prolactin-inhibiting factor (PIF). Endocrinology (submitted for publication).

16. Donovan, B.T. and J.J. Van der Werff ten Bosch. Physiology of Puberty. Williams and Wilkins: London, 216p, 1965.

17. Evans, J.S. and M.B. Nikitovitch-Winer. Reactivation of hypophysial grafts by continuous perfusion with median eminence extracts (MEE). Fed. Proc. 24:190, 1965.

18. Everett, J.W. Central neural control of reproductive functions of the adeno-hypophysis. Physiol. Rev. 44:373-431, 1964.

19. Gale, C.C., S. Taleisnik, H.M. Friedman and S.M. McCann. Hormonal basis for impairments in milk synthesis and milk ejection following hypothalamic lesions. J. Endocrinol. 23: 303-316, 1961.

20. Gittes, R.F. and A.J. Kastin. Effects of increasing numbers of pituitary transplants in hypophysectomized rats. Endocrinology 78:1023-1031, 1966.

21. Green, J.D. and G.W. Harris. Observation of the hypophysioportal vessels of the living rat. J. Physiol. (London) 108: 359-361, 1949.

22. Greenblatt, R.B. and V.B. Mahesh. Pituitary-ovarian relationships. Metabolism 14:320-326, 1965.

23. Greep, R.O. Physiology of the anterior hypophysis in relation to reproduction. IN: Sex and Internal Secretions, 3rd ed., Vol. I, 240-301, (W.C. Young, ed.) Williams & Wilkins, Baltimore, 1961.

24. Grosvenor, C.E. and C.W. Turner. Release and restoration of pituitary lactogen in response to nursing stimuli in lactating rats. Proc. Soc. Exp. Biol. Med. 96:723-725, 1957.

25. Grosvenor, C.E. and C.W. Turner. Assay of lactogenic hormone. Endocrinology 63:530-534, 1958.

26. Grosvenor, C.E., S.M. McCann and R. Nallar. Inhibition of nursing-induced and stress-induced fall in pituitary prolactin concentration in lactating rats by injection of acid extracts of bovine hypothalamus. Endocrinology 76:883-889, 1965.

27. Guillemin, R. Hypothalamic factors releasing pituitary hormones. Rec. Prog. Hor. Res. 20:89-121, 1964.

28. Halasz, B. and R.A. Gorski. Gonadotrophic hormone secretion in female rats after partial or total interruption of neural afferents to the medial basal hypothalamus. Endocrinology 80:608-622, 1967.

29. Harris, G.W. and D. Jacobsohn. Functional grafts of the anterior pituitary gland. Roy. Soc. (London), Proc., Ser. B. 139:263-276, 1952.

30. Harris, G.W. Sex hormones, brain development and brain function. Endocrinology 75:627-648, 1964.

31. Haun, C.K. and C.H. Sawyer, Initiation of lactation in rabbits following placement of hypothalamic lesions. Endocrinology 67:270-272, 1960.

32. Houssay, B.A., A. Biasotti, R. Sammartino. Modifications fonctionnelles de l'hypophyse après les lésions infundibulotubériennes chez le crapaud. Compt. Rend. Soc. Biol. 120:725-727, 1935.

33. Igarashi, M. and S.M. McCann. A new sensitive bioassay for follicle-stimulating hormone (FSH). Endocrinology 74:440-445, 1964.

34. Igarashi, M. and S. M. McCann. A hypothalamic follicle stimulating hormone-releasing factor. Endocrinology 74:446-452, 1964.

35. Kanematsu, S. and C.H. Sawyer. Effects of intrahypothalamic and intrahypophysial estrogen implants on pituitary prolactin and lactation in the rabbit. Endocrinology 72: 243-252, 1963.

36. Kanematsu, S. and C.H. Sawyer. Effects of hypothalamic and hypophysial estrogen implants on pituitary and plasma LH in ovariectomized rabbits. Endocrinology 75:579-585, 1964.

37. Kuroshima, A., Y. Ishida, C.Y. Bowers and A.V. Schally. Stimulation of release of follicle-stimulating hormone by hypothalamic extracts in vitro and in vivo. Endocrinology 76:614-619, 1965.

38. Lisk, R.D. Estrogen-sensitive centers in the hypothalamus of the rat. J. Exp. Zool. 145:197-208, 1960.

39. McCann, S.M. and H. M. Friedman. The effect of hypothalamic lesions on the secretion of luteotrophin. Endocrinology 67:597-608, 1960.

40. McCann, S.M., T. Graves and S. Taleisnik. The effect of lactation on plasma LH. Endocrinology 68:873-874, 1961.

41. McCann, S.M. and V.D. Ramirez. The neuroendocrine regulation of hypophyseal luteinizing hormone secretion. Rec. Prog. Hor. Res. 20:131-181, 1964.

42. McCann, S.M. and A.P.S. Dhariwal. Hypothalamic releasing factors and the nueorvascular link between the brain and the anterior pituitary. IN: Neuroendocrinology, Vol. I, 261-296, (L. Martini and F. Ganong, Eds.) Academic Press, New York, 1966.

S.M. McCANN, D.B. CRIGHTON, S. WATANABE, A.P.S. DHARIWAL, AND J.T. WATSON

43. McCann, S.M., A.P.S. Dhariwal and J.C. Porter. Regulation of the adenohypophysis. Ann. Rev. Physiol 30:589-640, 1968.

44. MacLeod, R.M., M.C. Smith and G.W. DeWitt. Hormonal properties of transplanted pituitary tumors and their relation to the pituitary gland. Endocrinology 79: 1149-1156, 1966.

45. Mittler, J.C. and J. Meites. In vitro stimulation of pituitary follicle-stimulating-hormone release by hypothalamic extract. Proc. Soc. Exp. Biol. Med. 117:309-313, 1964.

46. Mittler, J.C. and J. Meites. Effects of hypothalamic extract and androgen on pituitary FSH release in vitro. Endocrinology 78:500-504, 1966.

47. Moore, C.R. and D. Price. Gonad hormone functions, and the reciprocal influence between gonads and hypophysis with its bearing on the problem of sex hormone antagonism. Am. J. Anat. 50:13-71, 1932.

48. Nallar, R. and S.M. McCann. Luteinizing hormone-releasing activity in plasma of hypophysectomized rats. Endocrinology 76:272-275, 1965.

49. Nicoll, C.S. and J. Meites. Prolactin secretion in vitro effects of gonadal and adrenal cortical steroids. Proc. Soc. Exp. Biol. Med. 117:579-583, 1964.

50. Nikitovitch-Winer, M.B. Induction of ovulation in rats by direct intrapituitary infusion of median eminence extracts. Endocrinology 70:350-358, 1962.

51. Parlow, A.F. Bioassay of pituitary luteinizing hormone by depletion of ovarian ascorbic acid. IN: Human Pituitary Gonadotropins, 300-310, Albert, A., (ed). C.C. Thomas: Springfield, Ill., 1961.

52. Parlow, A.F. Differential action of small doses of estradiol on gonadotrophins in the rat. Endocrinology 75:1-8, 1964.

53. Parlow, A.F. IN: The Neuroendocrine Regulation of Hypophyseal Luteinizing Hormone Secretion, "Discussion", 171-181, McCann, S.M. and V.D. Ramirez. Rec. Prog. Hor. Res. 20:131-181, 1964.

54. Pasteels, J.L. Premiers résultats de culture combinée in vitro sécrétion de prolactine. Compt. Rend. Acad. Sci. 253:3074-3075, 1961.

55. Piacsek, B.E. and J. Meites. Effects of castration and gonadal hormones on hypothalamic content of luteinizing hormone releasing factor (LRF). Endocrinology 79:432-439, 1966.

56. Pfeiffer, C.A. Sexual differences of the hypophysis and their determination by the gonads. Am. J. Anat. 58: 195-225, 1936.

57. Ramirez, V.D. and S.M. McCann. Comparison of the regulation of luteinizing hormone (LH) secretion in immature and adult rats. Endocrinology 72:452-464, 1963.

58. Ramirez, V.D., R.M. Abrams and S.M. McCann. Effect of estradiol implants in the hypothalamo-hypophysial region of the rat on the secretion of luteinizing hormone. Endocrinology 75:243-248, 1964.

59. Ramirez, V.D., D. Moore and S.M. McCann. Independence of luteinizing hormone and adrenocorticotrophin secretion in the rat. Proc. Soc. Exp. Biol. Med. 118:169-173, 1965.

60. Ramirez, V.D. and C.H. Sawyer. Fluctuations in hypothalamic LH-RF (luteinizing hormone-releasing factor) during the rat estrous cycle. Endocrinology 76:282-289, 1965.

61. Ramirez, V.D. and C.H. Sawyer. Changes in hypothalamic luteinizing hormone releasing factor (LHRF) in the female rat during puberty. Endocrinology 78:958-964, 1966.

62. Ramirez, V.D., B.R. Komisaruk, D.I. Whitmoyer and C.H. Sawyer. Effects of hormones and vaginal stimulation on the EEG and hypothalamic units in rats. Am. J. Physiol. 212:1376-1384, 1967.

63. Rose, S. and J.F. Nelson. The direct effect of oestradiol on the pars distalis. Austr. J. Exp. Biol. Med. Sci. 35:605-610, 1957.

64. Rothchild, I. Relation of central nervous system, pituitary gonadotrophins, and ovarian hormone secretion. Fertil. and Steril. 13:246-258, 1962.

65. Schally, A.V. and C.Y. Bowers. In vitro and in vivo stimulation of the release of luteinizing hormone. Endocrinology 75:312-320, 1964.

66. Schally, A.V., T. Saito, A. Arimura, S. Sawano, C.Y. Bowers, W.F. White and A.I. Cohen. Purification and in vitro and in vivo studies with porcine hypothalamic follicle-stimulating hormone-releasing factor. Endocrinology 81:882-892, 1967.

67. Smith, E.R. and J.M. Davidson. Differential responses to hypothalamic testosterone in relation to male puberty. Am. J. Physiol. 212:1385-1390, 1967.

68. Smith, E.R. and J.M. Davidson. Positive and negative feedback actions of intrcerebral estrogen in prepuberal female rats. Fed. Proc. 26:366, 1967.

69. Steelman, S.L. and F.M. Pohley. Assay of the follicle stimulating hormone based on the augmentation with human chorionic gonadotrophin. Endocrinology 53:604-616, 1953.

70. Talwalker, P.K., A. Ratner, and J. Meites. In vitro inhibition of pituitary prolactin synthesis and release by hypothalamic extract. Am. J. Physiol. 205:312-218, 1963.

71. Wagner, J.W., W. Erwin and V. Critchlow. Androgen sterilization produced by intracerebral implants of testosterone in neonatal female rats. Endocrinology 79:1135-1142, 1966.

72. Watanabe, S. and S.M. McCann. Localization of FSH-releasing factor in hypothalamus and neurohypophysis as determined by in vitro assay. Endocrinology 82:664-673, 1968.

S.M. McCANN, D.B. CRIGHTON, S. WATANABE, A.P.S. DHARIWAL, AND J.T. WATSON

73. Watanabe, S., A.P.S. Dhariwal and S.M. McCann. Effect of inhibitors of protein synthesis on the FSH-releasing action of hypothalamic extracts in vitro. Endocrinology 82:674-684, 1968.

74. Worthington, W.C., Jr. Some observations on the hypophyseal portal system in the living mouse. Bull. Johns Hopkins Hosp. 97:343-357, 1955.

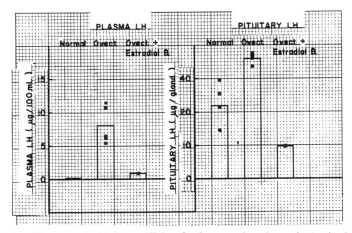

FIG. 1.   Plasma and pituitary LH levels in normal and ovariectomized rats;
the effect of estrogen on plasma and pituitary LH. Ovect. = ovariectomized;
Estradiol B. = estradiol benzoate. Dots represent values from individual
assays; the height of the bar gives the mean value. Values for LH are
expressed in terms of the N.I.H. ovine S-1 standard. (From McCann, S.M.
IN: Physiological Controls and Regulations. W.S. Yamamoto and J.R. Brobeck
(eds). W.B. Saunders Co.: Philadelphia, 1965.)

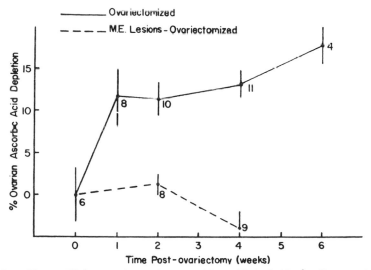

FIG. 2.   Plasma LH (per cent ovarian ascorbic acid depletion) after ovariectomy
of normal rats and those with median eminence lesions (constant diestrus). In
this and subsequent figures vertical lines indicate the SEM; the numbers give
the number of test rats used. (From Taleisnik, S. and S.M. McCann. Endocrinology
68:263, 1961.)

S.M. McCANN, D.B. CRIGHTON, S. WATANABE, A.P.S. DHARIWAL, AND J.T. WATSON

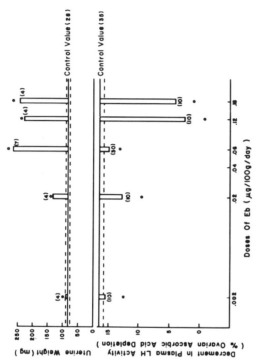

FIG. 3. Decrement in plasma LH and the increase in uterine weight produced by daily injections of estradiol benzoate (Eb) in ovariectomized females. (From McCann, S.M. and V.D. Ramirez. Rec. Prog. Hormone Res. 20:131, 1964.)

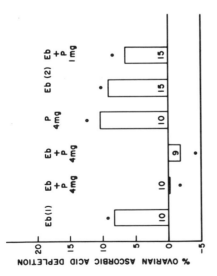

FIG. 4. Effect of progesterone (P) on plasma LH activity of ovariectomized rats pretreated with estrogen. Reading from left to right, each pair of columns represents the results of an experiment in which the LH activity of plasma from donors subjected to two different treatments was compared. The first two columns compare the plasma LH activity of donors pretreated with estradiol benzoate (Eb) only with that of another group treated with Eb followed by 4 mg of P. The next two columns compare the plasma LH activity of another set of donors given Eb followed by 4 mg of P with that of a group given only 4 mg of P. In the last two columns on the right, the LH activity in plasma of another group of donors given only Eb, as in the first experiment, is compared with that from a final group given Eb followed by 1 mg of P. (From McCann, S.M. Am. J. Physiol. 202:601, 1962.)

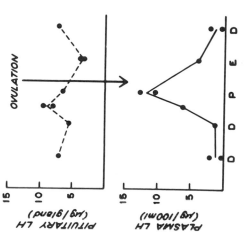

FIG. 5. Fluctuations in the hypophysial and plasma LH during the estrous cycle of the rat. The data for pituitary LH changes are from studies by Dr. Neena B. Schwartz at the University of Illinois. The data for plasma are those obtained in this laboratory. The letters on the abscissa refer to the days of the estrous cycle in the rat: D = diestrus; P = proestrus; E = estrus. (From McCann, S.M. Physiol. for Physicians 1 (#12):1, 1963.)

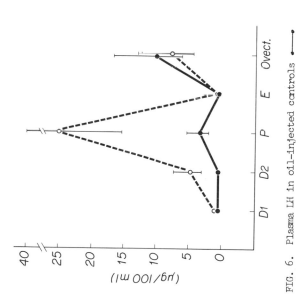

FIG. 6. Plasma LH in oil-injected controls ●——● and in rats injected with progesterone in oil ○– –○. Values are those for ovariectomized rats (ovect.) and those exhibiting 4 day estrous cycles. The dashed lines connect values for progesterone-treated rats, the solid lines represent the controls. Vertical lines indicate the 95 per cent confidence limits. D1 = diestrus, day 1; D2 = diestrus, day 2; P = proestrus; E = estrus.

S.M. McCANN, D.B. CRIGHTON, S. WATANABE, A.P.S. DHARIWAL, AND J.T. WATSON

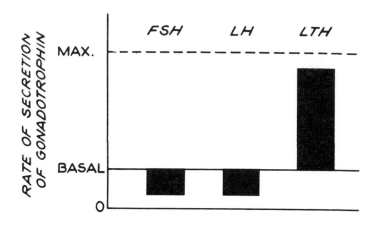

FIG. 7.   Effect of hypothalamic lesions on the secretion of the three gonadotrophins. Max = maximum. (From McCann, S.M. Physiol. for Physicians 1(#12):1, 1963.)

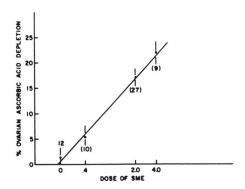

FIG. 8.   Effect of varying doses of stalk-median eminence extract (SME) on ovarian ascorbic acid depletion. Numbers on the abscissa refer to the number of hypothalami from which the extract was derived. Except for the control (0), the doses are on a log scale. From McCann, S.M. Am. J. Physiol. 202:395, 1962.)

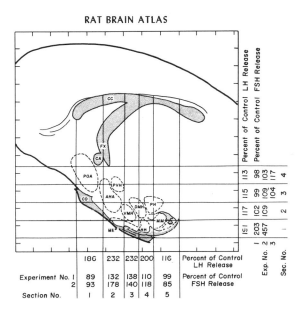

FIG. 9. Localization of FSH-RF and LH-RF as determined by horizontal and frontal sections. Key to abbreviations: CC = corpus callosum, FX = fornix, CA = anterior commissure, POA = preoptic area, CO = optic chiasm, AHA = anterior hypothalamic area, PVH = paraventricular nucleus, VMH = ventromedial nucleus, ME = median eminence, ARH = arcuate nucleus, DMH = dorsomedial nucleus, PH = posterior hypothalamic nucleus, MM = medial mammillary nucleus, CI = internal capsule, OT = optic tract, MFB = medial forebrain bundle, LHA = lateral hypothalamic area.

S.M. McCANN, D.B. CRIGHTON, S. WATANABE, A.P.S. DHARIWAL, AND J.T. WATSON

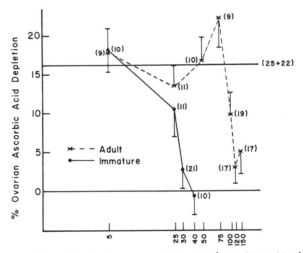

Log Dose Of Testosterone Propionate (μg./100gm./ day)

FIG. 10.   Decrement in plasma LH activity (per cent
ovarian ascorbic acid depletion) of castrated males
treated with testosterone propionate. (From McCann, S.M.
and V.D. Ramirez. Rec. Prog. Hormone Res. 20:131, 1964.)

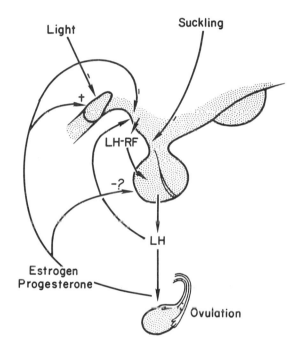

FIG. 11.   Diagram of the regulation of LH secretion.
+ = stimulatory effect, - = inhibitory effect.
Arrows point to the area where the effect is thought
to be mediated.

S.M. McCANN, D.B. CRIGHTON, S. WATANABE, A.P.S. DHARIWAL, AND J.T. WATSON

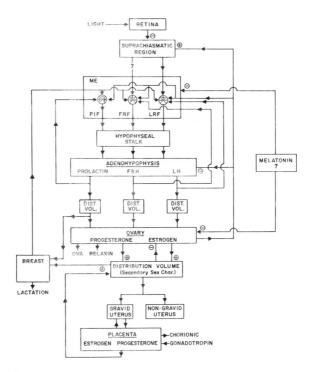

FIG. 12. Diagram of the regulation of the secretion of FSH, LH and prolactin. Melatonin, a compound synthesized by the pineal is shown as possibly inhibiting at the hypothalamic or ovarian level. This has yet to be proved. ME = median eminence region. Dist. Vol. = distribution volume.

NEENA B. SCHWARTZ
College of Medicine, University of Illinois, Chicago, Illinois

8. MODELING AND CONTROL IN GONADAL FUNCTION

INTRODUCTION

In the female mammal the function of the gonadal system, with its multiple components, is to deliver the ovum to the oviduct (i.e. ovulate) at the "right time". The right time is bounded by many considerations; time of day, time of year and ecological site all must be right in order for the male to be present and ready to mate, for fertilization to occur, for the fertilized ovum to be nurtured by properly prepared accessory sex structures within the female, and for the environment to be friendly and bountiful in order to permit survival of the young [1]. Ovulation must be carefully timed in relationship to all of the factors mentioned above because the ovum has a life span of only hours once it has been extruded from the ovarian follicle. A model of the mechanism by which this is accomplished in one species, the rat, is the subject of this paper.

There are a number of features of the gonadal system which will require inclusion in the model and which are so different from those in the previous systems considered in this volume that they should be mentioned at the outset of this discussion. First, there are three "gonadotrophic" hormones from the anterior pituitary which influence ovarian (target gland) function in different ways; the regulation of the secretion of each of these hormones is at least partially independent from that of the others. Second, the ovary secretes two hormones which have different effects on target organs, including the hypothalamo-pituitary axis. Third, the feedback actions of these ovarian hormones, which result in alterations in secretion rates of the pituitary hormones, are not monotonic, either as a function of dose of hormone or of time after hormone administration [5,38]. Fourth, as a result of the sequential action of the gonadotrophic hormones on the ovary an abrupt morphological change of state occurs. The transformation of follicles into corpora lutea (process of ovulation) (Figure 1); this morphological alteration is accompanied by a shift in the secretion rates of the two ovarian hormones.   Fifth, the system cycles at period lengths which are characteristic of different species; to neglect the cyclicity by choosing long time

NEENA B. SCHWARTZ

intervals for study in this system is to lose the essence of the function of the system.

It will be necessary to place certain restrictions on the domain of the model, at least at first. (a) In order to provide a model with enough detail to be useful, it will be necessary to restrict its applicability to one species. This is necessary because different relations exist in different species between the internal components of the system and various inputs from the environment; these differences establish the type of cycle which occurs and its period length. Accordingly, the present model will be restricted to the rat; a more general, but less detailed, model has been provided for a broad spectrum of mammalian species [27]. (b) The reproductive life of the rat can be displayed on a time scale which encompasses the entire life span of the animal (Figure 2). The phases of reproduction are listed in Table 1. The model will be restricted to a consideration of the events of the estrous cycle (Figure 2; Table 1-section IIA) and will not be scaled to include the stage of ontogenetic inductions, or senescence. (A later section of this chapter will return to these issues, and discuss how the model could be altered to represent the total life span). The events of interest in the study of the estrous cycle take place over four or five 24-hour day lengths. Within each 24-hour period many events of importance need to be included in the model; some recur regularly at a 24-hour interval (Figure 2) but others occur irregularly and on a shorter time scale (time constants of loss of hormones from the body, response times or delays of various tissues to hormones). (c) Finally, by isolating the female rat (and model!) from a male, the events of pregnancy need not be represented (Table 1-section IIB). Again, a later section of this chapter will indicate what elements need to be added to the model to permit pregnancy to be represented.

THEORIES OF THE ORIGIN OF CYCLICITY IN THE GONADAL SYSTEM

Three kinds of explanations have been offered to account for the remarkably regular and sustained repetition of events which constitutes the estrous cycle of the rat (Figure 2) and the reproductive cycles of other mammals as well. First, that the cycles are imposed from the outside by geophysical periodicities of various lengths. Second, that the periodicity resides in a given organ, which then becomes the pacemaker for the whole system. Third, that the periodicity resides in the interrelationships among the organ components and their parameters.

With respect to the period length of the estrous cycle in the rat, it is difficult to identify a geophysical event with a period of four or five days. Rats housed simultaneously in the same room show no synchrony of cycle stages, with 20 or

25% of the colony being in the same cycle stage on any given day. This indicates that
if an external event exists at these frequencies, it is serving as a determinant of
period length, but not as a synchronizer (unlike the 24-hour light-dark rhythm). Finally, it is possible to delay completion of the cycle by administering progesterone
for 7,8 or 9 days, starting on the morning after ovulation; under these circumstances
ovulation occurs during the fourth night after cessation of treatment regardless of
the number of injections [12]. It is as if the progesterone completely stops the system, which then resumes from the same point in each animal, although on different
days. These data argue against an absolute control of cycle stage from the outside.
(For that matter, the data also argue against the fuzzy hypothesis sometimes advanced
that the cycle is "inherent", thereby suggesting that period length is set by something in the body which is not subject to experimental study).

What then of the hypothesis that the cycle "resides" in one organ of the system?
The overt events of the rat estrous cycle which enable the investigator to follow the
sequence of stages are ultimately the result of estrogen and progesterone secretion
by the ovary, but removal of either the ovary or the pituitary gland will cause per-
manent cessation of these events. But so will a lesion placed properly in the hypothalamus, in the presence of an intact ovary and pituitary [2]. So far no one has
looked for a periodicity of four or five days duration in the activity of cells of
the central nervous system in the absence of an intact ovarian-pituitary axis, since
only in the presence of these latter organs is it possible to identify cycle stages.
Thus, while we can be reasonably certain that the cycle does not reside in the ovary-
pituitary complex, it could conceivably be located in neurons somewhere as yet un-
tapped.

The usual "explanations" of cyclicity in female reproduction, however, invoke
the interrelationships among the system components as the ultimate cause. When it
was recognized in the 1930's that hormones from the pituitary could stimulate ovarian
secretion and that the ovarian hormones could inhibit pituitary secretions, this simple system was labelled "push-pull" and it was considered sufficient to explain the
oscillations [14]. Lamport [14] and Rapoport [23] examined this hypothesis and found
it incapable, on mathematical grounds, of yielding sustained cycles. Rapoport suggested that: "More promise is held out by non-linear systems such as occur, for example, in relaxation oscillations. The fluctuations in such a system are due to more
or less abrupt passages from one steady state to another rather than to continuous
periodic changes in concentration". The models already presented in this volume for
the regulation of corticoid and thyroid hormone levels, which contain pituitary-tar-
get gland interactions similar to those initially proposed for the gonadal system,
are considered to yield steady-state solutions, and not to oscillate (except for
diurnal oscillations, which probably result from a diurnally changing signal provid-

NEENA B. SCHWARTZ

ing a continuous input to the system in question).

Danziger and Elmergreen [4] have provided a mathematical model of the menstrual cycle which is capable of oscillating because of an adjustment of system parameters so that two alternate solutions to a set of equations exist: the normal, unstable state when estrogen and progesterone negative feedbacks are too small to suppress totally the secretion rates of gonadotrophins from the pituitary; the degenerate, stable state, when the secretion rates of pituitary hormones become zero. While their model employs the concept of relaxation oscillations to produce cyclicity, as will also be the case in the present model, the system as modelled by Danziger and Elmergreen is so bare that is probably is not useful in describing the richness of the real system.

THE ESTROUS CYCLE IN THE RAT

The classical description of the estrous cycle in the rat was published in 1922 by Long and Evans [18]; their monograph is still not outdated because of the superbly detailed observations it contains. The most important technique one can use for detecting cycle stage in the rat remains the vaginal smear technique: a small sample of cells from the vagina is obtained daily and studied under the low power microscope. By this means one may detect the appearance of "cornified" epithelial cells which signify that estrogen secretion took place 24 or so hours earlier; on the morning of the day of cornified cells which precedes a morning of leukocytes, freshly ovulated ova can be detected in the oviduct. Rats exhibiting four-day cycles generally show only one morning when cells are cornified, while during five-day cycles two days of cornification is the more usual finding (Figure 3): on the morning labelled "estrus" cornified cells always appear in the smear. The "ballooning" of the uterus refers to the presence of fluid within the uterine lumen; this is also an excellent indicator of a preceding estrogen secretion and occurs only on the day of proestrus. Mating behavior, which also occurs only on the day of proestrus, is similarly a sign of preceding estrogen, and probably progesterone, secretion.

Until recently, most investigators spoke of the estrous cycle length in the rat as 4.5 days on the average, although even in the early data of Long and Evans [18] a distribution of cycle lengths reveals either four or five days as the most frequent periods. In the late 40's Sawyer and Everett [5] called attention to the fact that a given cycle was, in fact, either four days or five days in length and that in a particular rat one might observe "runs" of one cycle length, although it is the common experience of all workers in this field that a given rat may occasionally abruptly switch from cycles of one period length to the other, and back again.

The most important observation on the rat estrous cycle since the early monograph of Long and Evans came from the work of Everett and Sawyer [5] in which it was demonstrated that in rats housed under conditions of alternating light and darkness (lights on from 5AM to 7PM) and LH release responsible for the ovulation which terminates each cycle occurs after 2PM and before 4PM on the afternoon of proestrus (Figure 3). They demonstrated this by means of injections of inhibitory drugs such as the anesthetic barbiturates, or by timed hypophysectomy studies. Barbiturate injection or hypophysectomy at 2PM of proestrus prevented the ovulation expected that night; delay in treatment until 4PM permitted the ovulation to take place. With respect to the barbiturate injections a curious fact emerged: even though the anesthetic or sedative effects of the druge wore off after a few hours, ovulation was delayed in full 24 hours and could again be blocked by a repeated injection before 2PM the next day. Indeed, this could be shown for several days and suggested that an event was occurring in the system every 24-hours at 2PM. This hypothesis was strengthened when it was shown [5] that in the five-day cycle ovulation could be advanced 24 hours by an injection of progesterone on the morning of the second day of diestrus (Figure 3) and that this ovulation could also be prevented by drugs.

These experiments suggested two possibilities for regulation of the length of the estrous cycle [28]. The first is that every day the pituitary releases enough LH at 2PM to cause ovulation, but that the ovarian follicles are capable of responding only once every four or five days. If this were true, then cycle length would be determined by the response time of the ovary. The second hypothesis which fits the extant data equally well, is that the LH release does not occur every day, but only on the day of proestrus; however, some facilitatory event does occur every day at 2PM. A second event would then be necessary to trigger the release; normally these two events would occur only on the day which would then become proestrus. However, if ovulation were blocked by drugs at 2PM on proestrus, the second event would persist for another day. The obvious way to distinguish between these two hypotheses was to measure pituitary and plasma LH levels each day of the cycle. The results are summarized in Figure 4. It was clearly demonstrated that pituitary LH content fell and plasma LH rose only on the day of proestrus, thus lending support to the second hypothesis stated above.

Figure 4 also summarizes some other relevant data displayed on the time scale of the estrous cycle. FSH secretion by the pituitary also appears to occur on the afternoon of proestrus. LRF content in the hypothalamus drops acutely on this day and probably constitutes the immediate signal to the pituitary to secrete LH. What constitutes the stimulus to the hypothalamus? There is an increase in rate of progesterone secretion on the day of proestrus (Figure 4) but unfortunately none of the experimen-

NEENA B. SCHWARTZ

ters who measured this variable took into account the time of release of the LH (critical period) and so the data do not reveal whether progesterone secretion precedes the LH release, or follows it.

Our knowledge of estrogen secretion rates are all indirect, since this variable cannot at present be measured in small volumes of blood. The volume of individual follicles within the ovary shows a steady increase during the cycle and then an abrupt exponential increase after the ovulatory release of LH; when ovulation occurs, after midnight, the follicles disappear and new corpora lutea are formed (Figures 1,4). That estrogen secretion rates may to some extent reflect the increase in follicles volume, at least until the ovulatory surge of LH begins acting upon them, is suggested by the following information (used to construct the hypothetical estrogen secretion rate curve in Figure 4). (a) As was pointed out in the discussion of Figure 3, the ballooned uterus, mating behavior and vaginal cornification on the day of proestrus and estrus are positive signs of estrogen secretion within the last 24 hours or so, since each of these variables responds in exactly the same manner to the injection of estrogen into a rat from which the ovaries have been removed. (b) Removal of the ovaries from rats on the morning of the day before proestrus blocks all of these signs of estrogen secretion and also prevents the drop in pituitary LH content usually seen at estrus [26,34] (Figure 4). If the removal of the ovaries is delayed until the morning of proestrus all of these events occur normally. (c) Injection of single doses of an estrogen antagonist, MER-25 (which blocks the action of estrogen at receptor sites), also blocks the changes in the variables seen in Figure 3, including ovulation and LH release, when it is given on the diestrous day before proestrus [36]. Thus the evidence, albeit indirect, supports the hypothesis that estrogen secretion rates during the cycle follow a curve roughly as depicted in Figure 4; the evidence furthermore suggests that it may be the secretion of estrogen which is responsible for the LH release on the day of proestrus. We will tentatively conclude that the cycle is, in fact, due to the interaction of a daily input to the system signalling "time of day", occurring at 2PM, and a feedback signal from the ovary (estrogen?), both signals being necessary and sufficient to trigger the release of LH from the pituitary and, then, ovulation. This hypothesis is at the heart of the model to be presented.

Before proceeding to a description of the model the reader should note how few data points are displayed in Figure 4. This is due to the present extreme insensitivity of the methods, so that many rats are needed to provide each single bit of datum shown. And, of course, to insure synchronicity at the time of sacrifice, it is necessary to follow vaginal smears daily in each individial of a large group of rats for several weeks. Thus it is not surprising that the data points are so thinly distributed, but it does explain why our comparisons of the model and the real system at the present time must be more qualitative than quantitative.

DESCRIPTION OF THE MODEL FOR THE RAT GONADAL SYSTEM

The model is seen in Figure 5; it is the result of a collaborative effort with Dr. Joan C. Hoffman of the Department of Physiology, University of Rochester and has been previously described in brief [32]. Evidence for all the specific points (1) through (41) in the model can be found in References 2,5,7,9,19,20,24,27,32.

A number of elements have been omitted from the system as diagrammed in Figure 5. To keep the diagram from being unreadable, symbols have been omitted for the distribution, binding and metabolism of each of the secreted hormones; it should be understood that these symbols should lie between the secreting gland and the blood levels of the respective hormones. Similarly, symbols for the feedback transducer elements for E,P, dE/dt, dP/dt and LH are also omitted but are understood to be necessary before each comparator in Figure 5. The target organs for estrogen and progesterone, which constitute the accessory sex organs (vagina, uterus, oviducts) and secondary sex characters (emitted odors, neuromuscular apparatus for displaying mating behavior, etc.) have been omitted from the model in order to avoid the necessity of accepting inputs from these factors. In a later section the consequences of permitting reentry to the model from some of these factors will be discussed. Finally, in the model seen in Figure 5 we have deliberately side-stepped the issue of where the steroid feedbacks are acting (hypothalamus, anterior pituitary gland or elsewhere) by omitting the symbols for the hypothalamic releasing (LHFR, FRF) and inhibiting (PIF) factors. These factors are just regarded as one unspecified form of signal in the input pathways to the pituitary in the model.

In the model the ovary is represented to the right, the pituitary in the center and "central" factors to the left. In general, the left hand side can be thought of as the central nervous system, except for some feedbacks which occur at the level of the pituitary gland itself. In Figure 5 the numbers represent the following: (1) FSH and LH cause follicle growth and estrogen secretion (2); this is the so-called "folliculotrophic" action of the gonadotrophins on the ovary. Progesterone secretion may occur during the preovulatory phase also (3). (4) LH also induces ovulation when it is presented to the "ripe" follicle; as a result estrogen secretion stops (5) and a corpus luteum is formed (6). (This process was illustrated in Figure 1 as it appears in the real system). Two opposing inputs influence the life-span of the corpus luteum and its ability to secrete estrogen and progesterone (9): a "leuteotrophic" stimulus and a "luteolytic" inhibitory mechanism. For the rat, prolactin

NEENA B. SCHWARTZ

is luteotrophic (7) and LH may be luteolytic (8). During the normal rat cycle prolactin is not secreted, so that this part of the system ((7), (8), *9)) is inoperative; prolactin release occurs only when mating takes place and thus ensures an active set of corpora lutea. This point will be discussed again later.

Before discussing the other parts of the model two general comments are necessary. The pituitary gland and its secretory output of LH are represented twice in order to indicate that the model hypothesizes two subsystems which can control the synthesis and release of LH. It should be understood that the same gland is simply receiving inputs from two functionally (and probably anatomically) separate units. Furthermore, synthesis and release rates are represented separately for LH since changes in pituitary LH content (storage) occur under various non-steady state conditions. While for the system as a whole it is only the release rate which is important, changes in content have been easier to determine because of the relative insensitivity of the methods for measuring plasma levels of the hormones; these changes in content have been important in detecting changes in the system (as seen in Figure 4).

K_1 (10) is the input or setpoint for LH synthesis rate (13). LH synthesis rate can be lowered by estrogen in the blood (11) in a negative feedback relationship; there is also some evidence that LH levels in the blood may likewise exert a negative influence on LH synthesis (12). Points (14) through (17) represent similar influences on LH release rate. The subsystem just described (10-17), plus the ovarian follicle (1-3), constitute the complete "folliculotrophic" subsystem. Progesterone feedback probably does not influence this system.

Points (18) to (41) constitute the "surge" subsystem; it is responsible for the release of the ovulatory surge of LH which results in ovulation at (4) (see Figures 3 and 4). A 24-hour clock is shown (18) which provides an input, K_2 and K_2', at 2PM to the surge system at (19) and (20). This input, plus an input from changing estrogen (22) and/or progesterone (23) concentration in the blood, interact ((21) and (24)) and ((31) and (30)) to yield a positive signal at (25) and (32), ultimately yielding increased LH synthesis (29) and release (36). The synthesis and release of the ovulatory surge can be blocked by high levels of circulating estrogen ((26), (33)), progesterone ((28), (35)) and perhaps by LH itself ((27), (34)). Three other influences on the surge subsystem are also shown: (37) chronic progesterone injection or secretion can alter the timing of release of the ovulatory surge of LH; (38) barbiturates can block release of LH and ovulation: (39) to (41) cervical stimulation can sometimes induce release of LH and ovulation.

A number of sequelae of long term treatment, or approximately steady-state inputs, are predictable from the model. Removal of the anterior pituitary (hypophysectomy) results in complete absence of ovarian secretion, cessation of follicular growth and absence of ovulation, effects which are clearly in line with the model. Removal of both ovaries causes, within a week, high plasma levels of LH and FSH, as well as high pituitary contents of these hormones. This occurs, in terms of the model (Figure 5), as the consequence of abolition of the estrogen negative feedback at (11) and (15), leading to the unopposed input to the system of K_1 and K_1'.

The model also predicts that, in the absence of estrogen or progesterone secretion, the surge sub-system would cease to function since it is dependent on simultaneous inputs from the derivative of one or the other of these steroids, plus the "clock" input. It is not easy to test this hypothesis experimentally, since the ovarian secretions and their effects on accessory sex tissue (vagina, etc.) are the usual criteria of cycle stage. One experiment we have carried out which provides a first approximation to investigating this important point was to remove the ovaries and to wait until high amounts of LH accumulated in the plasma and pituitary. We then asked whether these values show a 24-hour periodicity and, if so, whether release of LH into the plasma would occur during the same time period as on the day of proestrus (Figure 4) in the intact rat. The experimental data are shown in Figure 6. Both pituitary and plasma LH values are much increased over normal (during the cycle pituitary LH content shows maximal values of about 10μg, and plasma LH is undetectable except during the critical period for LH release on proestrus). Pituitary LH content showed no significant variation over the 24-hour time period; however, plasma LH was significantly lower in the afternoon and evening and showed a significant rise when the lights went on at 5AM. If this system were showing the same critical period seen in the cycle (Figure 4) the highest plasma LH values would have been found between 2-3PM and 6-7PM. Thus, these data provide presumptive evidence that the surge subsystem may not operate in the absence of the ovary, and that the folliculotrophic system may itself show a 24-hour periodicity.

Whereas we have just seen the difficulty of examining the surge subsystem in the absence of the folliculotrophic system, the converse situation proves to be more easily attainable experimentally. A priori one would predict from the model that if the surge subsystem were removed from operation, with retention of the folliculotrophic system, a steady state of estrogen, FSH and LH secretion would result, with absence of ovulation. This does appear to happen in three different situations which lead to a phenomenon called "persistent estrus", because the rat stops cycling and shows uterine and vaginal signs of continuous estrogen secretion.

The first of these situations is induced by injection of the male sex hormone into the female within the first five days of birth [19]. If the dose is high enough,

NEENA B. SCHWARTZ

the female never cycles but shows persistent estrus, in spite of a normal ovary and pituitary. We may hypothesize that the male hormone has permanently cancelled out the surge system at some point, with only the folliculotrophic steady-state system remaining in operation. Estrogen secretion is constant, as shown by the continuous vaginal cornification, and the pituitary is still able to respond to removal of the ovary by increasing LH synthesis and release, as would be predicted from the model.

The second procedure which can lead to a steady-state of estrogen secretion is the placing of a lesion in the anterior part of the hypothalamus. In fact, just separating the anterior hypothalamus from the central area by a knife-cut can cause this [8]. Presumably this causes an anatomical isolation of the surge subsystem at some place along the pathway to the pituitary.

There is yet a third technique for inducing persistent estrus in the rat, which is perhaps the most interesting since the animal itself does not need to be directly manipulated. The model (Figure 5) indicates that in order for the LH surge to be triggered two conditions are necessary and sufficient: it must be the right time of day and there must be a changing concentration of estrogen or progesterone. Removal of the clock signal, then, ought also to lead to a steady state of estrogen secretion. It has been known for years that keeping a rat in constant light eventually causes persistent estrus, but not immediately. A priori, there is some difficulty with predicting exactly what might happen to gonadal function since exposing an animal to constant light does not remove the near-24 hour periodicity inherent in many other variables,but simply takes them out of phase with the outside world. Thus, there appears to be an endogenous periodicity of each sub-unit within the animal which is not exactly 24 hours in length, but may be a little longer than this, or a little shorter. So it might be predicted that ovulation would not stop in constant light but might occur at odd hours. Previous studies on reproduction in continuous light or continuous darkness have emphasized the results obtained after a number of weeks of exposure [11] and have not examined the transients (time scale=days) in the system. We have placed rats in continuous light and sampled gonadal function throughout a 120 day period. The results are summarized in Table 2.

During the first 30 days in continuous light many animals continued to show cyclic changes in vaginal cornification, uterine ballooning, ovulation (Figure 1) and pituitary LH content. However, the events were desynchronized, since pituitary LH content did not always correspond to ovulation, and uterine ballooning and vaginal cornification did not always indicate the days of proestrus and estrus (Figure 3), as far as ovarian morphology was concerned. These data suggested that the various organs do each have their own endogenous near-24 hour rhythms and were pulling apart timewise without an external timer. During the second stage (Table 2), persistent estrus developed, and this was occasionally interrupted by ovulation. Pituitary LH

levels were preovulatory, in general. This stage appears to represent further de-
synchronization, with the pituitary and ovary badly out of phase and not able to respond at the right times. Finally, however, the system does appear to go into a per-
manent steady state with high plasma LH, low pituitary LH, steady estrogen secretion,
and no ovulation. In this stage, it appears that there is no clock functioning, or
that events have become hopelessly desynchronized, or that constant light has had a
harmful effect on some component of the system, aside from the lack of a timing signal.
In terms of our real data, then, the model (Figure 5) is adequate in having only one
clock represented, since each organ undoubtedly has its own rhythm. But as long as
there is an external synchronizer in the form of an alternating light-dark environment,
each component is operating at the right time and the model is correct.

Thus far in our comparisons of the model in Figure 5 with experimental data we
have examined the consequences of experimental situations as seen some days after the
onset of treatment. But it has also proved possible to carry out some perturbations
at specific times during the cycle and examine the immediate effects on the variables
(Figure 3,4) within a 48 hour period. The perturbations used were barbiturate injection, ovary or pituitary removal, injection of the estrogen antagonist MER-25, or injection of antibodies to LH or FSH. The initial set of experiments was performed before the critical period for LH release on the day of proestrus, thus examining the
surge subsystem; the second set of experiments, using the same inputs, was carried out
on the day before proestrus, examining the folliculotrophic subsystem postulated as
causing ovarian secretion and follicular growth (Figure 5).

Table 3 summarizes the experimental procedures tested on the day of proestrus.
Since ovariectomy itself at 10AM does not prevent the estrous vaginal cornification,
it is not surprising that some of the other procedures can do so. Ovariectomy also
did not prevent the estrous drop in pituitary LH content, implying that the estrogen
necessary for this, as well as for the vaginal cornification, had already been secreted by 10AM. Ovulation is blocked by hypophysectomy at 2PM, but not at 4PM, delin-
eating the critical period for the ovulatory surge of LH. Barbiturates injected before the critical period block ovulation and LH release (high pituitary LH and low
plasma LH) for only 24 hours. (FSH release (Figure 4) is simultaneously inhibited by
barbiturates [21]. Anti-LH-serum given before the critical period also blocks ovulation but permits LH depletion from the pituitary; ovulation is then delayed at least
one whole cycle length. Anti-FSH-serum appears to have no effect on the LH release
for ovulation or the ovulation itself, but does appear to delay the appearance of
ovulation in the following cycle.

The results summarized in Table 3 can be placed within the context of the model
(Figure 5). The fact that ovary removal on the morning of proestrus does not prevent
LH release suggests that by that time the surge subsystem has already responded to

dE/dt. This may mean that the components involved take some time to respond to changing estrogen levels, but continue to retain a state of facilitation even after blood levels of estrogen drop with ovariectomy. The hypophysectomy experiments simply define the time of the critical period. The barbiturate experiments also delineate this time (since it can be shown that barbiturate injection after 4PM does not prevent ovulation) but in addition they demonstrate that the ovulation blockade is the result of failure of release of the ovulatory surge of LH from the pituitary. What permits the ovulation to occur 24 hours later? There are signs in the barbiturate-blocked rat that estrogen secretion is prolonged, since vaginal cornification and uterine ballooning may persist an extra day [5,26]. Thus, in terms of the model (Figure 5), the barbiturates acted somewhere in the surge system at (38) to prevent LH release and termination of estrogen secretion at (5); estrogen levels continued to rise, and by the next day when the critical period occurred again at (18) dE/dt has again acted at (22). Unlike the barbiturates, anti-LH-serum blocks ovulation for at least one cycle; moreover, there are no signs of persistence of estrogen secretion. In model terms (Figure 5), the antibodies are reacting with LH which has already been released (i.e., the surge system has fired) and prevents ovulation by blocking at (4); however, the anti-LH-serum also blocks LH from acting at (1) and thus estrogen secretion stops. Thus there is no signal at (22) to retrigger the surge system the next day, or indeed, until the next crop of follicles begins secreting estrogen.

The effects of the same perturbations imposed on the day before proestrus are summarized in Table 4. The effects of ovariectomy or administration of MER-25 early on this day are to remove all signs of estrogen secretion (uterine ballooning and mating behavior, as well as vaginal cornification); postponement of these two procedures until late in the day permits the necessary estrogen to be secreted. Failure of release of the ovulatory surge of LH, as a result of estrogen removal on this day, is also suggested (Table 4). (The MER-25 also blocks the FSH depletion from the pituitary at estrus [21]. The hypophysectomy experiments reveal that pituitary secretion must precede ovarian secretion. Barbiturates do not prevent estrogen secretion. Anti-LH-serum on diestrus, but not anti-FSH-serum, prevents estrogen secretion.

These results may also be interpreted in terms of the model (Figure 5). The data suggest that on the day before proestrus the folliculotrophic subsystem is activated, since there is evidence that both the ovary and the pituitary must be in situ for at least part of the day for the events of proestrus and estrus to occur. Barbiturates apparently do not affect this system, since they do not block estrogen secretion. The anti-LH-serum must be acting at (1) in Figure 5 to prevent action on the ovary of the LH. Anti-FSH-serum had no effect on estrogen secretion, as it had failed to affect ovulation (Table 3). These results suggest that the release of FSH which takes place on the afternoon of proestrus (Figure 4) does not influence the crop of follicles destined to ovulate that night, but may be responsible for initiating development of the next crop of follicles (see Figure 4, follicle volume). In this respect the model is inadequate because it should represent two crops of follicles, and separate the effects of the secreted LH and FSH on these. Since the data on anti-FSH-serum are so recent, the interpretations just made are perhaps premature; accordingly, the model was not revised to include what may turn out to be fanciful speculations.

EXPANSION OF THE DOMAIN OF THE MODEL

In order to expand the model to include ontogenetic changes (Table 1) it would be necessary to include a timing device scaled to the life span of the rat with inputs to the model in Figure 5 at various points. During the first five days or so of the life span the surge sub-system (Figure 5) is susceptible to the male hormone, testosterone. As discussed in a preceding section, injected testosterone will cancel this system and create steady-state conditions in the folliculotrophic system. This is the normal state in the male. Thus, the areas of the nervous system which contain the surge sub-system are inherently female and under normal circumstances during the life of the female are not subjected to androgens. To make the model complete, our life span clock should temporarily permit androgens, if present, to suppress permanently the LH surge for ovulation by removing the possibility of inputs at (19) and (20) in Figure 5. Incidentally, by including the life span clock for both the early "inductions", such as androgen action, as well as the puberty shift, the model in Figure 5 becomes a fair approximation to regulation of LH secretion in the male rat, if the testis is substituted for the ovary.

There is evidence [20] that before puberty less estrogen (per body weight) needs to be injected to inhibit pituitary LH release, than after puberty. Prepubertally, LH secretion and estrogen secretion are both kept to extremely low levels, so that the accessory sex tissue remains in the immature state. This suggests that the two inputs of the folliculotrophic system, K_1 and K_1', are low and thus only slight stimulation of the pituitary occurs, and low estrogen levels are effective in suppressing LH secretion. Supporting this hypothesis is the observation that the immature rat can still respond to ovary removal by increasing plasma LH levels [17,20]. Thus puberty might result when the clock mechanism which alters with the life span changes the values of K_1 and K_1' to the higher setpoint values seen during the adult estrous cycle.

Senescence in the female rat is characterized by a gradual development of persistent estrus, suggesting that the life span clock may gradually change the sensitivity of some element in the surge system so that eventually the system ceases operation. Parenthetically, in the human female menstrual cycles are less regular just

NEENA B. SCHWARTZ

after puberty and near menopause (which results from ovarian failure) than during the middle reproductive years [37].

In order to incorporate pregnancy into the model in Figure 5 four basic additions must be made: (a) In order to obtain mating behavior, the estrogen and progesterone output arrows on the right of the diagram should be shown activating the mating behavior center in the hypothalamus; (b) cervical stimulation, shown at (39), must enter the model so as to trigger prolactin secretion; (c) sperm must gain access to the ovum (seen as a terminal output in the follicle in Figure 5), and fertilization take place; (d) the uterus must be represented in the model, in order to show implantation of the fertilized, dividing ovum and the subsequent production of the placental organ. A possible model of prolactin secretion resulting from cervical stimulation has already been presented [27]. Prolactin secretion probably starts immediately after mating and continues for nine days or so; it activates the corpora lutea to secrete large quantities of progesterone (Figure 5 at (17)). Meanwhile the estrogen and progesterone from a new set of follicles, or the corpus luteum secretion, prepare the uterus for implantation. Implantation occurs on the fifth day after ovulation and mating; the next ovulation is blocked because the corpora lutea are producing enough progesterone to prevent the LH surge (progesterone blocks this system at (28) and (35) in Figure 5). Once implantation of the dividing ovum has taken place a new organ, the placenta, is formed which secretes a gonadotrophin which has luteotrophic activity. This gonadotrophin then substitutes for the prolactin from the pituitary, and maintains the secretory capacity of the corpora lutea until the end of pregnancy (22 days or so). Thus the maintenance of pregnancy is dependent on progesterone secretion from the ovary throughout, but is independent of the pituitary gland after 12 days in the rat, because of the formation of a new, temporary organ, the placenta, which substitutes for the pituitary. In a sense, the pregnant rat is a persistent estrous rat, since the folliculotrophic system remains intact, while the surge system is suppressed by progesterone. This concept of pregnancy has recently been discussed in more detail [35].

QUANTITATION OF THE MODEL

The model of gonadal function in the rat (Figure 5) is only a model of the real system in a qualitative sense even with the modifications suggested in the representation of FSH secretion, the inclusion of ontogenetic time clocks and of the components necessary for the representation of pregnancy. What of a quantitative nature can be said about this system?

The important variables which have been measured as a function of time during the cycle were summarized in Figure 4, in nondimensionalized form. The cited references contain the original data expressed in actual units of measurement. It has already been pointed out that the insensitivity and expense of our current methodology is the cause of the scarcity of data. With the new immunoassay methods for the protein pituitary hormones, and the possibility of some newer techniques for the ovarian steroid hormones, more data should accumulate rapidly.

Some of the parameters of the system have also been measured. Gay and Bogdanove [6] have estimated, in rats lacking ovaries, that the half life of LH is 28 minutes and that the plasma LH levels are 0.1 µg/ml (but may fluctuate during the 24 hour day (Figure 6)); correcting this for plasma volume and recalculating on the basis of 24 hours yields 37.4 µg/rat/day for the value of K_1 in Figure 5. This is the daily LH release rate in the absence of estrogen feedback. Similar measurements yield half-life values for FSH of 120 minutes and plasma levels of 11 µg/ml; the "setting" for FSH is therefore 960 µg/rat/day. The half-life of estrogen in the rat is about 30 minutes [13]; estimates from other species would suggest that the half life for progesterone is closer to 60 minutes. The amount of LH released in the ovulatory surge is estimated to be about 15 µg [31].

Very little information is available to permit the calculation of feedback parameters; that is, to express the secretion rates of FSH and LH (or prolactin) in terms of plasma levels of estrogen, progesterone, FSH or LH. Injection of a single dose of 1 mg of progesterone at the right stage of the cycle can induce ovulation [38] but repeated injections of progesterone will inhibit ovulation [24]. Similarly, estrogen in a single injection of 50 µg can induce ovulation by triggering the release of the ovulatory surge of LH, but repeated injections of much smaller amounts can inhibit LH release, ovulation and also follicle growth [5,7,20]. These experimental observations are represented in the model (Figure 5), but do not lead to any immediately useful quantitative expressions, since the plasma levels of estrogen or progesterone at which these feedback effects occur are not yet known. One potentially useful relationship which emerges from data such as these is that plasma estrogen levels are probably 2 or 3 orders of magnitude below progesterone levels, based on the relative amounts which exert feedback actions, and also on relative levels necessary to exert effects on accessory sex tissue.

Three sets of transfer functions occur in the whole system: (a) gonadotrophic hormone secretion as a function of the hypothalamic releasing or inhibiting factors; (b) ovarian secretion and ovulation as a function of gonadotrophic hormones; (c) accessory sex tissue growth and functional capacity as a function of ovarian hormones. Tripling the dose of pig LHRF almost doubles the amount of LH released from the pituitary of the rat [25]; there is an amplification factor suggested since increasing the dose of LHRF from .05 to .15 µg increases LH secretion from 1.0 µg to 1.6 µg.

NEENA B. SCHWARTZ

(It should be recognized that expressions of amounts of the pituitary hormones are all relative to standard preparations and have no absolute meaning in terms of molecular equivalence at the present time). Measuring the transfer functions of the ovary has been difficult not only because of difficulty in measuring the steroids, but also because the organ itself probably undergoes changes in transfer function from stage to stage in the cycle, as morphology changes (Figure 1). In addition to these inherent difficulties a factor which has contributed heavily to a lack of pertinent information has been the interest of most investigators in the intermediate pathways of steroid synthesis, rather than in the overall end-products. As a result no data are available at present which yield information, in the rat, concerning the rates of ovarian secretion of estrogen or progesterone as a function of LH and/or FSH levels in the ovarian arterial blood. What is known is that both hormones are necessary, simultaneously or sequentially, for estrogen secretion [5,7]. Once the ovarian follicles have been brought to the correct degree of ripeness, about 15 µg of LH can induce ovulation [31]. The transfer functions of the uterus, mammary tissue, vagina and mating behavior centers in terms of estrogen and progesterone have been much more throughly studied than those of the ovary or pituitary, but since these organs do not appear in the model at present, they will not be discussed.

SUMMARY

Let us summarize by reexamining the rat estrous cycle (Figures 3,4) using the model (Figure 5). On the morning of estrus there are freshly ovulated ova in the oviduct because of the LH released the day before. The FSH released at that same time initiates the growth of a new crop of follicles. It takes some time for the ovary to respond to this FSH, and the folliculotrophic LH being secreted, as the result of low estrogen feedback. Each day a facilitation signal from the biological clock clicks in at the appropriate time. By the day before proestrus, follicles are secreting estrogen at a high rate and possibly also some progesterone. The ovarian steroids begin acting at some central point, and on the day which becomes proestrus, dE/dt and possibly dP/dt have become high enough so that when the daily facilitation starts, the ovulatory subsystem gets triggered and a surge of LH is released. This causes ovulation and terminates estrogen secretion. When ovulation occurs the follicles disappear and corpora lutea are produced. At the same time a new crop of follicles starts up because of the FSH and if the corpora lutea are not made to secrete by prolactin secretion, another cycle starts.

The model shown here is not a simple push-pull system, but perhaps can be characterized as a "push-pull-click-click" system. There are two sequential relaxation oscillations postulated: the first one is the abrupt release of LH from the pituitary when the surge subsystem fires (Figure 5-(32)) and the second is the abrupt conversion of the follicles into corpora lutea (Figure 5-(4), (6)), with a cessation of estrogen secretion (Figure 5-(5)). These two abrupt events permit initiation of the next cycle. Ovulation occurs at a specific time of day, by means of the clock mechanism; but the day on which this occurs depends on the derivative feedback signal from the ovary which indicates that the follicles are capable of responding (Figure 5-22)).

If the model is correct we can see that a cycle length of four and a half days would be impossible, since release of the LH surge must occur at 24 hours intervals. What causes some cycles to be four days in length and some to be five (Figure 3)? The simplest hypothesis suggested by the model is that the rate of rise of estrogen feedback is too slow in the five-day rat and thus does not achieve the necessary rate of change of the steroid feedback by the critical period on the fourth day of the cycle. A complete 24 hours would then have to elapse before another critical period occurs at which time LH release could be triggered. This explanation does in fact seem to have some validity, since in five-day cycles estrogen levels appear to rise more slowly, as seen by a delay in the proestrous uterine weight increase (Figure 3) and by some comparative timing studies carried out with the estrogen antagonist in four-day and five-day cycles [36]. Thus it appears that estrogen levels do not rise high enough, soon enough, to set the surge system in motion on the 4th day and thus LH release is delayed and a five day cycle results. Additional evidence suggests that the steroid secretion itself is not delayed by a full 24 hours but only by a fraction of this period. As a consequence, the duration of the estrogen secretion is actually prolonged in the five-day cycle [12]. This is again predictable from the model (Figure 5), since the 24 hour delay in LH release prevents the termination of estrogen secretion until the fifth day. At present we do not know what causes the slow rate of estrogen secretion; it could be the result of delayed pituitary folliculotrophin secretion, or slow responsivity of the ovary.

In spite of the scarcity of quantitative information, the model in Figure 5 has had heuristic value in interpreting experimental data and in designing new experiments. It appears to offer a reasonably satisfactory explanation of the estrous cycle in the rat and to take into account many of the distinguishing peculiarities of the pituitary gonadal system in this species, and in others. One inverse measure of the success of a model is its "half-life"; the more provocative and the more testable a model the shorter must be its time constant. As we have seen, the model in Figure 5 is probably already out-dated by newer data from our own and other laboratories. From this model, more complete models will evolve which should approach more and more closely the magnificient richness of the reproductive system in that most useful and fertile of mammals, the laboratory rat.

NEENA B. SCHWARTZ

ACKNOWLEDGMENTS

I would like to express my gratitude to Mr. William L. Talley for his consistently excellent technical assistance; to the staff of the Aeromedical Laboratory for the environmentally controlled animal housing they have provided; and to the Endocrinology Study Section of the National Institutes of Health for supplies of NIH-LH and NIH-FSH used as standard preparations in the published and unpublished studies reported here. Unpublished work was supported by research grants from National Institutes of Health, GRSG 184 and HD 00440, and the University of Illinois Graduate College Research Fund.

TABLE I

PHASE OF REPRODUCTION IN THE FEMALE RAT

I.   PRE-ADULT
     Ontogenetic Inductions -
          Early pre and post natal "organization"
          Prepuberal events
          Puberty

II. ADULT
     A.   Cyclic, non-pregnant -
          Follicle growth-estrogen (progesterone) secretion
          Behavioral estrus
          Ovulation
          (Activation of corpus luteum or "pseudopregnancy"; luteolysis)

     B.   Pregnant -
          Mating and fertilization
          Implantation
          Placenta-gonadotrophin secretion
          Delivery
          Lactation

III.   SENESCENCE

TABLE II

SEQUENCE OF EVENTS IN CONTINUOUS LIGHT

	STAGE I	STAGE II	STAGE III
Duration of Cont. Light	5-30 days	≤ 60 days	> 60 days
Ovulation	Cyclic	Occasional	Absent
Vag. smear	Cyclic	Predom. Cornified	Cornified
Uterus	Cyclic	High (proestrus)*	High (Proestrus)*
Pit. LH	Cyclic (High→Low)	High (proestrus)	Low (Estrus)
Plasma LH	Cyclic (High→Low)	"High"*	"High"*
Synchrony of Above Variables	Asynchronous	?	?

TABLE III

EXPERIMENTAL PROCEDURES TESTED ON DAY OF PROESTRUS

Procedure	Time	Events at Estrus* Vag.	Ova	Pit. LH	Next Cycle	Reference
NONE	–	C	YES	LOW	NORMAL	5,26,28
OVAX	10AM	C	–	LOW	NONE	26
HYPOX	2PM	C	NO	–	NONE	5
HYPOX	4PM	C	YES	–	NONE	5
BARB	2PM	C	NO	HIGH	OVA-24 HRS.	5,26,33
ANTI-LH	1PM	C	NO	LOW	DELAY	30,31
ANTI-FSH	1PM	C	YES	?	DELAY	30

Table II. * Uterine weight, and plasma LH content, are in a steady state in Stages II and III.
            Reference [16].

Table III. * Next Morning
           ? Not tested as yet

NEENA B. SCHWARTZ

TABLE IV

EXPERIMENTAL PROCEDURES TESTED ON THE DAY BEFORE PROESTRUS

		Events at Estrus*			Next	
Procedure	Time	Vag.	Ova	Pit. LH	Cycle	References
NONE		C	YES	LOW	NORMAL	5,26,28
OVAX	10AM	L	–	HIGH	NONE	26
OVAX	8PM	C	–	?	NONE	15
MER-25	10AM	L	NO	HIGH	DELAY	36
HYPOX	12N	L	NO	_	NONE	15
HYPOX	3PM	C	NO	–	NONE	15
BARB	10AM-4PM	C	YES	LOW	NORMAL	33
ANTI-LH	11AM	L	NO	?	?	30
ANTI-FSH	11AM	C	YES	?	DELAY	30

REFERENCES

1. Amoroso, E.C. and F.H.A. Marshall. External factors in sexual periodicity. Marshall's Physiology of Reproduction Vol. 1, part 2, pp. 707-831, 1960.

2. Bogdanove, E.M. The role of the brain in the regulation of pituitary gonado-tropin secretion. Vitamins and Hormones 22: 205-260, 1964.

3. Boling, J.L., R.J. Blandau, A.L. Soderwall and W.C. Young. Growth of the Grafian follicle and the time of ovulation in the albino rat. Anat. Record 79: 313-331, 1941.

4. Danziger, L. and G.L. Elmergreen. Mathematical models of endocrine systems. Bull. of Math. Biophysics 19: 9-18, 1957.

5. Everett, J.W. The mammalian female reproductive cycle and its controlling mech-anisms. in Sex and Internal Secretions, (W.C. Young, ed.) Vol. 1, 3rd. Ed., pp. 497-555, Williams and Wilkins Co., Baltimore, 1961.

6. Gay, V.L. and E.M Bogdanove. Observations on the clearance of endogenous LH from the plasma of previously castrated rats. Fed. Proceedings 26: 533, 1967; also personal communication.

Table IV   * Two Mornings Later
             ? Not tested as yet

7. Greep, R.O. Physiology of the anterior hypohysis in relation to reproduction. in Sex and Internal Secretions, (W.C. Young, Ed.) Vol. 1, 3rd. Ed., pp. 240-301, Williams and Wilkins Co., Baltimore, 1961.

8. Halasz, B. and R.A. Gorski. Gonadotrophic hormone secretion in female rats after partial or total interruption of neural afferents to the medial basal hypothalamus. Endocrinology 80: 608-622, 1967.

9. Harris, G.W. and B.T. Donovan. (eds) The Pituitary Gland. 3 volumes. University of California Press, Los Angeles, 1966.

10. Hashimoto, I. and R.M. Melampy. Ovarian progestin secretion in various reproductive states and experimental conditions in the rat. Fed. Proceedings 26: 485, 1967; and personal communication.

11. Hoffmann,J.C. Effects of light deprivation on the rat estrous cycle. Neuro-endocrinology 2: 1-10, 1967.

12. Hoffmann, J.C. and N.B. Schwartz. Timing of ovulation following progesterone withdrawal in the rat. Endocrinology 76: 626-631, 1965.

13. Jensen, E.V. and H.I. Jacobson. Basic guides to the mechanism of estrogen action. Rec. Prog. Hormone Research. 18: 387-414, 1962.

14. Lamport, H. Periodic changes in blood estrogen. Endocrinology 27: 673-680, 1940.

15. Lawton, I.E. and C.H. Sawyer. Timing of gonadotrophin and ovarian steroid secretion at diestrus in the rat. Endocrinology 82: 831-836, 1968.

16. Lawton, I.E. and N.B. Schwartz. Pituitary-ovarian function in rats exposed to constant light: a chronological study. Endocrinology 81: 497-508, 1967.

17. Lawton, I.E. and N.B. Schwartz. A circadian rhythm of LH secretion in ovariectomized rats. Am. J. Physiol. in press.

18. Long, J.A. and H.M. Evans. The oestrous cycle in the rat and its associated phenomena. Mem. Univ. Calif. 6: 1-148, 1922.

19. Martini, L. and W.F. Ganong (ed.) Neuroendocrinology (2 volumes) Academic Press, N.Y. 1966.

20. McCann, S.M. and V.D. Ramirez. The neuroendocrine regulation of hypophyseal luteinizing hormone secretion. Rec. Prog. Hormone Research 20: 131-181, 1964.

21. McClintock, J.A. and N.B. Schwartz. Pituitary FSH content in cyclic female rats. Fed. Proceedings 26: 366, 1967; also unpublished observations.

22. Ramirez, V.D. and C.H. Sawyer. Fluctuations in hypothalamic LH-RF (luteinizing hormone-releasing factor) during the rat estrous cycle. Endocrinology 76: 282-289, 1965.

23. Rapoport, A. Periodicities of open linear systems with positive steady states. Bull. Math. Biophysics 14: 171-183, 1952.

NEENA B. SCHWARTZ

24. Rothchild, I. Interrelations between progesterone and the ovary, pituitary, and central nervous system in the control of ovulation and the regulation of progesterone secretion. Vitamins and Hormones 23: 209-327, 1965.

25. Schally, A.V., C.Y. Bowers, W.F. White and A.I. Cohen. Purification and in vivo and in vitro studies with porcine luteinizing hormone-releasing factor (LRF). Endocrinology 81: 77-87, 1967.

26. Schwartz, N.B. Acute effects of ovariectomy on pituitary LH, uterine weight, and vaginal cornification. Am. J. Physiol. 207: 1251-1259, 1964.

27. Schwartz, N.B. Newer concepts of gonadotropin and steroid feedback control mechanisms. in J.J. Gold (ed) Textbook of Gynecologic Endocrinology Pub.-Hoeber Medical Division, Harper and Row, New York, pp. 33-50, 1968.

28. Schwartz, N.B. and D. Bartosik. Changes in pituitary LH content during the rat estrous cycle. Endocrinology 71: 756-762, 1962.

29. Schwartz, N.B. and D. Calderelli. Plasma LH in cyclic female rats. Proc. Soc. Exp. Biol. Med. 119: 16-20, 1965.

30. Schwartz, N.B. and Charles Ely. Unpublished observation.

31. Schwartz, N.B. and J.J. Gold. Effect of a single dose of anti-LH-serum at proestrus on the rat estrous cycle. Anat. Rec. 157: 137-149, 1967.

32. Schwartz, N.B. and J.C. Hoffmann. A model for the control of the mammalian reproductive cycle. Excerpta Med. Int. Cong., No. 132, 997-1003, 1967.

33. Schwartz, N.B. and I.E. Lawton. Effects of barbiturate injection on the day before proestrus in the rat. Neuroendocrinology 3: 9-17, 1968.

34. Schwartz, N.B. and W. Talley. Effect of acute ovariectomy on mating in the cyclic rat. J. Reprod. and Fert. 10: 463-466, 1965.

35. Schwartz, N.B. and W. Talley. Daily measurement of pituitary LH content during pregnancy in the rat: J. Reprod. and Fert. 15: 39-45, 1968.

36. Shirley, B. J. Wolinsky and N.B. Schwartz. Effects of a single injection of an estrogen antagonist on the estrous cycle of the rat. Endocrinology in press.

37. Treloar, A.E., R.E. Boynton, B.G. Behn and B.W. Brown. Variation of the human menstrual cycle through reproductive life. Int. J. Fertility 12: 77-126, 1967.

38. Zeilmaker, G.H. The biphasic effect of progesterone on ovulation in the rat. Acta Endocrinologica 51: 461-468, 1966.

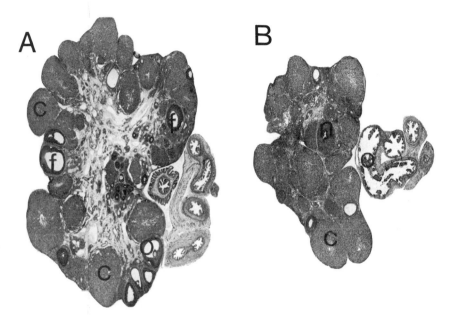

FIGURE 1. Sections of ovaries (magnification 10X) from two rats running estrous cycles. (These two rats were maintained in continuous light and were showing the fifth cycle in that environmental condition when the ovaries were removed. The ovaries are indistinguishable from those removed from rats housed under alternating light-dark conditions.) A. Proestrus. C=corpora lutea from previous ovulations. f=ripe follicles destined to ovulate that night. O=ovum in follicle. B. Estrus. C=corpora lutea from previous ovulations. n=newly formed corpus luteum. O=three ova are visible in this section of the oviduct. (These photographs are taken from Reference [16].

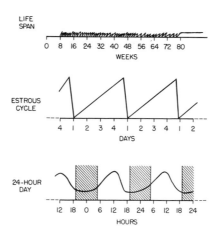

FIGURE 2.   Time scales for reproductive events
in the female rat. The ordinates do not represent specific variables, but are simply designed
to illustrate that there are variables which
change during time periods.

Timing of Events in the Rat Estrous Cycle

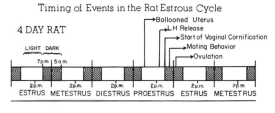

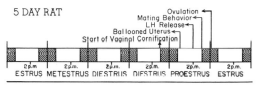

FIGURE 3.   The timing of events in the rat estrous cycle.
The figure summarizes the naming of the days of the cycle
and the events which are accepted as occurring on these
days. As can be seen, the day of proestrus is well
delineated by many variables. The day of estrus can also
be distinguished easily by the vaginal cornification which
is inevitably visible in the morning, as well as by the
freshly ovulated ova seen in the oviduct (Figure 1B).

NEENA B. SCHWARTZ

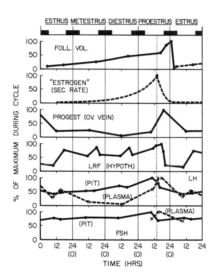

FIGURE 4. A number of variables seen in the
time scale of the four-day cycle. The vertical
dotted line on the day of proestrus denotes 2PM.
The data have been recalculated, on the basis
of the maximum (100%) seen during the cycle,
from the following references: follicle volume
[3]; "estrogen" secretion rate [26,34,36];
progesterone in the ovarian vein blood [10];
LRF in the hypothalamus [22]; LH in the
pituitary and plasma [20,26,28,29]; FSH in
the pituitary and plasma [21].

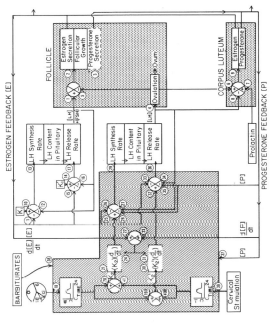

FIG. 5. A model representing the control of luteinizing hormone synthesis and release in the female rat. The inputs designated by K or K¹ are assumed to be greater thar cr equal to zero. A detailed description appears in the text. This figure appeared originally in Reference [32].

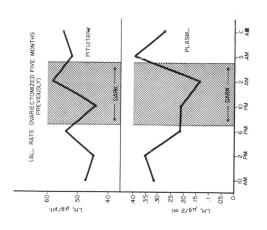

FIG. 6. Pituitary and Plasma LH over 24-hour Day.

WILLIAM F. GANONG
School of Medicine, San Francisco Medical Center, University of California, San Francisco, California

9. BRAIN-ENDOCRINE INTERRELATIONS: AN OVERVIEW

INTRODUCTION

The material I wish to present in this paper is of two types. The first gives a broad review of brain-endocrine relationships, pulling together some of the things that are discussed in the preceeding pages of this volume and adding some comments about areas for future research. The second is a presentation of some pertinent new data from my own laboratory which is included to illustrate the points being made and to update previously published work. Also, I had originally planned to include some philosophical comments on control systems and endocrine function. However, it seems to me that such general questions are adequately covered in the preceeding pages of this volume, and I think that anyone reading these pages will achieve a greater appreciation of the virtues, the limitations and the potential of modeling and the modeling approach in endocrinology.

Let me introduce the subject of brain-endocrine relationships and of homeostatic mechanisms in general by showing a diagram (Fig. 1); this is obviously a diagram rather than a model. It is important in thinking about regulatory processes in the body to analyze them in terms of sensors that respond to perturbations in the internal or external environment, integrating systems that process the information from the sensors, and effector organs that bring about changes which help the animal to adjust to the environment.

The two great integrating systems in the body are the endocrine system and the nervous system, and recent research has demonstrated that in most instances they work together to control endocrine function. However, the nervous system is not always involved. In some situations, the sensor, the integrator and the effector are all located within the endocrine gland itself. For instance, a decline in the amount of calcium in the circulation acts directly on the parathyroid glands to in-

256

crease the secretion of the parathyroid hormone [20]. This increased parathyroid hormone secretion raises the circulating calcium level, thereby shutting off the stimulus which initiated the increased secretion. Conversely, a rise in the circulating calcium level decreases parathyroid secretion. A high calcium level also acts on another group of endocrine cells which secrete the calcium-lowering hormone called calcitonin. In nonmammalian vertebrates, calcitonin is apparently secreted by the ultimobranchial bodies, a pair of small glands of previously unknown function. In mammals, the ultimobranchial bodies have become incorporated into the thyroid gland, where they form the so-called clear cells. A rise in plasma calcium apparently acts directly on the calcitonin secreting cells to increase their secretion. Thus, the plasma calcium level is defended by two negative feedback control mechanisms involving two different hormones.

In instances in which the nervous system is the integrator involved in the control of endocrine function, the multiple inputs from the sensors that relay information to the brain become available to modify endocrine function. The effectors available to the nervous system are summarized in Fig. 2. In addition to skeletal muscle, which after all is the "final common pathway" for all behavior, the classical effectors include smooth muscle and the exocrine glands. To these must now be added the endocrine glands that are under neural control. Indeed, a large segment of the endocrine system is actually an effector arm of the nervous system. The endocrine organs that are regulated at least in part by the nervous system are listed in Table 1.

TABLE I
Hormones whose secretion is regulated at least in part by the nervous system.

Hormone	Endocrine Organ
insulin	pancreas
norepinephrine	adrenal medulla
epinephrine	
vasopressin	
oxytocin	
α MSH	
β MSH	
ACTH	pituitary
TSH	

BRAIN-ENDOCRINE INTERRELATIONS

GH
FSH
LH
prolactin

CRF
TRF
GHRF
FSHRF   hypothalamus
LRF
PIF

BRAIN-PANCREAS RELATIONSHIPS

Notice that the list includes the insulin-secreting cells of the pancreas. The major control of insulin secretion is, of course, a direct feedback of the circulating blood-glucose level on the beta cells of the pancreatic islets, and the precision with which the insulin level follows the blood glucose level is remarkable. However, branches of the right vagus nerve innervate the beta cells, and it has been demonstrated that stimulation of these nerve fibers can bring about insulin secretion irrespective of the blood glucose level at the particular moment. The physiological role of this vagal system is debated, but certain investigators feel it plays a role in functional hypoglycemia [21]. This is a syndrome that occurs in tense, hard-driving individuals and is characterized by episodes in which the blood glucose falls to low levels. The hypoglycemia deprives the brain of glucose which leads to even more tension and nervousness.

The adrenergic as well as the cholinergic division of the autonomic nervous system appears to affect insulin secretion. Cahill [1] has pointed out that epinephrine has the ability to inhibit insulin secretion, and beta adrenergic stimulators appear to be able to stimulate insulin secretion. In addition, a number of gastrointestinal hormones stimulate insulin secretion, and secretion of these hormones is partially regulated by neural mechanisms. Secretin has this capacity and so does pancreozymin. Glucagon also stimulates insulin secretion, and at least in some species, glucagon appears to be secreted from the gastrointestinal tract as well as the pancreas. Thus, there are many variables that affect insulin secretion. Fortunately, one can perfuse the isolated pancreas and measure insulin output while changing these variables one at a time. Research of this type is providing interesting insights into the details of the secretion process [11].

BRAIN-ADRENAL MEDULLA RELATIONSHIPS

The adrenal medulla is another gland under neural control. It secretes epinephrine, norepinephrine and small quantities of other substances. It is a gland which lends itself to experimental study because one can cannulate the adrenal vein and measure its hormone output directly. Its secretory cells are innervated by preganglionic autonomic fibers from the nervous system. Indeed, the adrenal medullary cells are in effect postganglionic neurons which have lost their axons and become specialized for secretion directly into the blood stream. This relationship is summarized in Fig. 3, which also emphasizes the endocrine character of many different types of neurons. Neurons are endocrine organs in the sense that they liberate chemical substances at their endings. In the case of motor neurons, acetylcholine is liberated. In the autonomic nervous system, acetylcholine is liberated at preganglionic endings and either norepinephrine or acetylcholine is liberated at postganglionic endings. In the hypothalamus, the releasing factors secreted into the portal vessels control anterior pituitary secretion, and in the posterior pituitary, vasopressin and oxytocin are secreted by neurons into the general circulation.

It appears that the adrenal medulla has received little attention from those interested in constructing models, partly because much of its input is open loop. A wide variety of sensory stimuli increase adrenal medullary secretion. However, there is also a closed loop negative feedback regulation between adrenal medullary secretion and the blood glucose level. Hypoglycemia is a potent stimulus to adrenal medullary secretion (Fig. 4), and the epinephrine which is secreted works along with other factors to raise the blood glucose level, shutting off the stimulus.

Some years ago, we* began a search for the location of the integrating center involved in this feedback loop. In our studies of adrenal medullary secretion [2],

---

* Incidentally, when I say "we", I am talking about a variety of associates and students. I was thinking the other night that as one goes on in science, the meaning of the term "we" undergoes a progressive change. When the young professor fresh out of postdoctoral training says "we", he really means "I did it", but he's being polite. There then comes a period when "we" means the professor and his students, and this is followed by a period when "we" means the students and the professor. Finally, the time arrives when "we" means the students did it, and the professor went to a symposium to talk about it. Suffice it to say that in this presentation, I am leaning heavily on the work of a group of very excellent students and postdoctoral fellows.

BRAIN-ENDOCRINE INTERRELATIONS

we first transected the midbrain. Disconnecting the forepart of the brain from the
rest of the nervous system in this fashion failed to abolish the response to hypoglycemia (Fig. 5). Therefore, the center where the response is integrated must be
caudal'to the midbrain. We next cut the spinal cord, and found the response still
remained intact (Fig. 6). On the other hand, cutting the adrenal nerves abolished
the response. Therefore, the neural integrating center must be located in the spinal
cord. Subsequently, we were able to abolish the response by taking out a small segment of the spinal cord (Fig. 7). It should be pointed out that Crone has performed
similar experiments in sheep and finds that cord section does block the response to
hypoglycemia [4]. There are some stimuli such as acidosis [3] which act directly on
the adrenal gland, and the possibility that our cord sectioned dogs became acidotic
due to hypotension cannot be completely excluded. However, it seems likely that we
have identified a neuroendocrine control mechanism that is integrated in the spinal
cord.

BRAIN-HYPOTHALAMUS-PITUITARY RELATIONSHIPS

Another gland regulated by the nervous system is the pituitary. This small
organ actually secretes at least ten hormones. Six hormones are secreted by the
anterior lobe of the pituitary: ACTH, TSH, growth hormone, FSH, LH and prolactin.
Two melanocyte stimulating hormones, α and β MSH, are secreted by the intermediate
lobe. The posterior lobe secretes oxytocin and vasopressin. These ten hormones
have extremely widespread effects in the body, and consequently, it is hardly surprising that the pituitary gland is often called the conductor of the endocrine
symphony.

Anterior pituitary secretion is under hypothalamic control by means of a group
of releasing factors and related substances secreted into the portal vessels. The
chemistry of these factors is a matter of debate at the moment, but the evidence for
their existence seems incontrovertible [16]. The principal factors are summarized
in Fig. 8. As indicated in this figure, current evidence indicates that nerve fibers from a variety of locations end on the capillary loops from which the portal
vessels arise, and the portal vessel system transmits the factors directly to the
anterior pituitary. Notice that there are five releasing factors plus a factor that
inhibits prolactin secretion; prolactin is subject to inhibitory rather than stimulatory control by the brain. I might add that this particular figure was prepared
about one year ago as an illustration for a textbook, and the field moves so fast
that it is already out of date. For instance, it does not contain McCann's growth
hormone inhibiting factor. However, it remains a first order approximation to the

truth.

One additional comment about the anterior pituitary is in order. An easy and accurate radioimmunoassay for growth hormone in small volumes of plasma is now available, and with it, minute to minute sampling can be done. Furthermore, we have considerable information about the feedback loops involved in the control of growth hormone secretion. Therefore, I suggest that the mechanism regulating growth hormone secretion is one which commends itself to the modeling approach, and I look forward to rapid advances in this field.

Secretion of the MSH's by the intermediate lobe is probably under hypothalamic control. Not shown in Fig. 8 are an MSH-stimulating factor and an MSH-inhibiting factor reportedly found in the hypothalamic extracts. However, there is also evidence that MSH-secreting cells are innervated, and that these nerve fibers control MSH secretion. In addition, nobody really knows what the MSH's do in mammals; they have established functions only in amphibia and reptiles. Only future research can resolve the enigma of intermediate lobe function and control in mammals.

The posterior lobe hormones are a different matter. Here, details of the mechanisms regulating secretion are known. The control of oxytocin secretion provides a typical example. The principal action of oxytocin is on muscle-like cells lining the ducts in the breasts. Contraction of these cells causes milk to squirt into the cisterns behind the nipple, and from there it passes to the exterior. If the breasts contain milk, the action of oxytocin is, therefore, the release of milk to the exterior.

What controls the secretion of this posterior pituitary hormone? There are many touch receptors around the areola and nipple of the breast, and stimulation of these touch receptors sets up impulses which enter the spinal cord. These impulses eventually enter the reticular formation in the midbrain and funnel into the hypothalamus, where they stimulate the paraventricular nucleus. The axons of the stimulated paraventricular neurons then liberate oxytocin into the general circulation. This is a unique example of a neuroendocrine feedback mechanism. The infant suckling at the breast stimulates the tactile receptors, oxytocin is secreted, and the milk is squeezed out cafeteria-style into the waiting mouth of the infant.

The regulation of vasopressin secretion is even more interesting and pertinent from the modeling point of view. Two facts about vasopressin are important in the present context. The first is that vasopressin acts on the kidney in such a way that it causes retention in the body of water in excess of solute. The hormone makes the urine become more concentrated than the blood plasma, and this makes the plasma and other body fluids more dilute. In the absence of vasopressin, the urine becomes more dilute than the blood. Water is lost in excess of solute, and the con-

BRAIN-ENDOCRINE INTERRELATIONS

centration of solute - i.e., the osmolality - of the plasma rises. Thus, by adjusting the rate of vasopressin secretion, the concentration of solute in the body fluids can be adjusted. The second point about vasopressin is that it is a hormone manufactured by and secreted by neurons. The neurons are located primarily in the supraoptic nuclei of the hypothalamus, and their axons end in the posterior pituitary. Stimulation of these neurons causes vasopressin to be secreted into the circulation.

The principal input to the supraoptic neurons is information about the osmolality of the plasma. When the osmolality rises, receptors sensitive to this parameter are stimulated, and they in turn stimulate the supraoptic neurons. The osmoreceptors are in all probability located in the anterior hypothalamus and possibly in the supraoptic nuclei themselves. At any rate, the resultant increase in circulating vasopressin leads to dilution of the body fluids, shutting off the stimulus which initiated the increased vasopressin secretion. Conversely, if the body fluids become dilute, as they are to do after one drinks water or attends a cocktail party, vasopressin secretion is inhibited. There is a diuresis and the body fluids become more concentrated until normal osmolality is again achieved. Thus, osmotic control of vasopressin secretion is a classic example of a continuous, active feedback mechanism monitoring and defending the osmolality of the body.

There is also a volume input to the supraoptic neurons. When the blood volume declines, there is an increase in vasopressin secretion, and when blood volume is greater than normal, vasopressin secretion is reduced. The receptors that sense the changes in blood volume are partly in the walls of the great veins and atria of the heart, and they are stimulated when these structures are distended by an increased volume of blood within them. However, a decrease in blood volume also lowers the blood pressure, and this decreases the discharge rate of the carotid and aortic baroreceptors. These receptors in the carotid sinuses and aortic arch are in effect stretch receptors, and it is important to note that when the blood pressure rises, their rate of discharge increases; conversely, a fall in blood pressure is associated with a decrease in discharge rate. Since a decrease in blood pressure is associated with an increase in vasopressin secretion, the input from these receptors must inhibit the secretory mechanism.

Notice the possibilities for interaction between these two control systems. Suppose for instance, that one has chronic hypovolemia, for one reason or another, or that the receptors have been fooled into thinking such hypovolemia exists. In this situation, the osmoreceptor mechanism would be expected to act as if its setpoint had been altered to defend a lower than normal plasma osmolality. This happens in a variety of clinical diseases, and the result is a chronic reduction in plasma osmolality with the production of a number of untoward symptoms.

The vasopressin-secreting cells are neurons, and a variety of afferent fibers end on them. Thus, it is not surprising to find that the vasopressin mechanism also has an open loop aspect. Emotional stimuli, pain, and stressful stimuli increase vasopressin secretion. Increases are also produced by a variety of drugs. Pain and drugs cause increased secretion to occur in patients who have had surgical operations. In postoperative patients, the osmoreceptor is in effect reset and hypotonicity of considerable magnitude can actually develop.

These examples illustrate the interaction of closed and open loop components in the control of vasopressin secretion. As far as I know, the system has not been looked at by the modelers, and it seems to me that it is a system which commends itself to a careful analysis from this point of view.

OTHER BRAIN-ENDOCRINE INTERACTIONS

There are many other brain-endocrine interactions. For instance, neuroendocrine interrelationships play a key role during development. Gorski has pointed out that the brain is either male or female in the pattern of its regulation of pituitary secretion [10]. The inherent brain pattern is female, and in genetic males, it is exposure to a small quantity of androgen early in life that makes the pattern male. If for any reason the male hormone does not come along, the male pattern does not develop and one has in effect a female brain in a male body. Conversely, if the brain in a genetic female is exposed to male hormone during the critical period, one has in effect a male brain in a female body.

Another instance of effects of hormones on development is the brain-pituitary-thyroid interaction which Etkin believes triggers metamorphosis in frogs [5]. Sexual behavior and related behavioral patterns are greatly affected by hormones in lower animals, and at least modified by hormones in man. The gonadal hormones act on the brain to unlock stereotyped instinctual patterns of sexual behavior. Thus, brain-endocrine interactions are multiple, complex and fascinating.

SENSITIVITY ASPECTS OF ENDOCRINE FUNCTION

There are some specific aspects of feedback control in the endocrine system that deserve special comment. The first of these is the variation in the sensitivity of secretory organs that is produced by their prior history. Liddle [15] has pointed out that ACTH has two actions on the adrenal; it stimulates the secretion of glucocorticoid hormones by the adrenal and it conditions the adrenal so' that it is more responsive to subsequent doses of ACTH. If ACTH is taken away, the adrenal becomes less responsive and puts out less hormone per unit of ACTH reaching

BRAIN-ENDOCRINE INTERRELATIONS

it. This decline is illustrated in Fig. 9, which shows that 8 days after hypophysectomy in the dog, adrenal responsiveness to ACTH is less than one-fifth what
it is four hours after hypophysectomy. The converse is seen, for instance, in
patients who have had surgical operations. The ACTH secreted during surgery makes
the glands of these patients more responsive, and for some days postoperatively,
their glucocorticoid responses to ACTH are increased. Yates has argued [22] that
this sensitivity change had a time constant of days, and consequently could be ignored in his model. However, I am not sure that this conclusion is completely correct. In a rat, there is a clearly measurable decrease in adrenal sensitivity within 24 hours after hypophysectomy [6], and Perkoff and associates showed that in
normal humans [19], there is a significant diurnal fluctuation in the sensitivity
of the adrenal gland to ACTH. Therefore, the time constant of the sensitivity change
must be of the order of hours rather than days.

Fluctuations in the sensitivity of other hormone-secreting cells also occur.
You will recall that in addition to glucocorticoids, the adrenal glands secrete
aldosterone and sex hormones. We have found that fluctuations in the sensitivity
of the aldosterone secreting portion of the adrenal occur independent of fluctuations
in the sensitivity of the glucocorticoid secreting portion. Figure 10 shows the
sensitivity of the adrenal in dogs fed a normal sodium intake. The dogs were acutely
hypophysectomized and nephrectomized, then injected with graded doses of ACTH. The
open bars show the resulting increments in the output of 17-hydroxycorticoids, an
index of the output of one of the principal glucocorticoids. The black bars show
the increments in aldosterone secretion. Output of 17-hydroxycorticoids reaches a
maximum with as little as 10 milliunits (mU) of ACTH, but it takes almost 100 mU to
cause a significant increase in aldosterone secretion. In animals fed a low sodium
diet, the pattern of secretion is different (Fig. 11). After just 5 days of the low
sodium diet, as little as 10 mU of ACTH stimulates aldosterone secretion. Secretion
of 17-hydroxycorticoids is not changed. The shift is even more marked after 14 and
30 days on the diet (Fig. 12). There is a similar shift in the sensitivity to angiotensin II [7]. Thus, a low sodium diet makes the aldosterone-secreting mechanism
selectively more sensitive to the stimulatory effects of angiotensin II and ACTH
without changing the response of the 17-hydroxycorticoid-secreting mechanism to
these two hormones (Fig. 13). We have been able to show that the change produced by
a low sodium diet is due to chronic stimulation of the adrenal by renin, or more
specifically, by the angiotensin II generated by the high renin level in the dogs
on the low sodium diet. Conversely, a high sodium diet makes the aldosterone-secreting mechanism less sensitive, presumably by inhibiting renin secretion. Thus,
not only the glucocorticoid-secreting portion of the adrenal, but also the al-

dosterone-secreting portion has a memory; i.e., its response is determined by its past history. The same appears to be true in the case of the juxtaglomerular cells, the endocrine "organ" which secretes renin. In Fig. 14, the rise in plasma renin produced by hemorrhage in normal dogs is compared to that produced in dogs fed a low sodium diet for 14 days. Not only is the control value higher, but the rise is much greater in the dogs fed the low sodium diet. Thus, it appears that in modeling the endocrine system, it is going to be essential to build in a variable or variables to account for the past secretory history of the organ being modeled.

Another sensitivity change which **deserves** consideration is the one which McCann [17] talked about yesterday: the change in hypothalamic sensitivity which appears to underlie the development of puberty. Puberty is a remarkable phenomenon. In all species of mammals of which I am aware, the young are born in a sexually immature state, and they undergo a period of growth and development before their sexual organs mature and they begin to reproduce. The termination of the sexual development process we call puberty. What is it that holds back the gonadotropin-secreting mechanism until the proper age, or alternatively, what is it that turns on the gonadotropin-secreting mechanism at the proper age? This is a question to which more and more investigators are addressing themselves. The normal failure to mature before the appointed age is not a deficiency at the gonadal level, since one can demonstrate that the gonads are responsive to injected gonadotropic hormones. There are gonadotropins in the pituitary gland before puberty, so it is not a deficiency in the gonadotropins themselves. In addition, the gonadotropins in the anterior pituitaries of the immature animals can be secreted in the proper environment. Harris and Jacobson [12] showed this when they transplanted the pituitary glands of immature animals into the pituitary fossa of mature female rats, and found that as soon as the blood supply was reestablished, estrus cycles reappeared. Interestingly enough, this was true whether the grafted pituitary was from a male or female; thus, the pituitary gland is sexless and it is the sex of the brain that determines the pattern of pituitary secretion.

Another possible explanation of lack of sexual development in young animals would be a deficiency of the hypothalamic-releasing factors necessary for stimulation of gonadotropin secretion. However, the necessary releasing factors are present prepubertally. McCann has presented data showing that luteinizing hormone releasing factor (LRF) is present [17], and Kragt and Dahlgren in my laboratory [13] have demonstrated the presence of follicle stimulating hormone releasing factor (FSHRF) as well.

McCann has presented a hypothesis about the mechanism responsible for puberty which is widely held, and which I think has a good deal of evidence to support it.

BRAIN-ENDOCRINE INTERRELATIONS

This is the view, that in immature animals, the hypothalamus is very sensitive to the negative feedback effects of gonadal steroids, and that the small amounts of circulating gonadal steroids in young animals hold back gonadotropin secretion. According to this view, puberty is precipitated by a decline in the sensitivity of the feedback mechanism in the hypothalamus. This permits secretion of gonadotropin to occur.

Secretion of gonadal hormones certainly starts very early in life. Baker and Kragt in my laboratory have studied secretion of these hormones in immature animals. I would like to present their data, because I think it shows clearly the temporal pattern of secretion, and also because it shows what good data can sometimes be obtained with very simple techniques. What Baker and Kragt did was to remove the ovaries of rats at birth and follow the development of one of the principal ovarian target organs, the uterus. The results are shown in Fig. 15. There was some growth of the uterus in the absence of the ovaries. However, there was greater growth of the uterus in the presence of the ovaries from 10 days of age on, and, even at 5 days of age, there is a difference in weight even though it was not statistically signif- icant. Puberty occurs in female rats at 35-40 days of age. Baker and Kragt also studied male rats. Removal of the testes at birth led to significantly slower growth of the ventral prostate and the seminal vesicles, two organs maintained by androgen in the adult (Fig. 16). Thus, in both male and female rats, there appears to be an appreciable secretion of gonadal steroids as early as the 5th-10th day of life.

Kragt [14] has also studied the FSH content of the pituitary in rats at various ages. In females, the content rises to a peak and then drops off (Fig. 17). Data from the literature on LH content are also shown in Fig. 17. In males, FSH content rises to a peak at 20-30 days of age and then stays high (Fig. 18). Total gon- adotropin content has been reported to fall, so the fall must be due to a decline in LH content. The value of measuring pituitary hormone content by itself is limited, but when content is placed in the context of the rate of gonadal secretion, gonadal and sexual accessary organ weight, and the hypothalamic content of FSHRF, it is of considerable interest. We are currently unable to measure blood levels of gon- adotropins in immature animals, but this may become possible in the near future.

When during development does negative feedback of gonadal steroids on the hypo- thalamus first appear? Baker and Kragt addressed themselves to this problem by the simple device of taking out one ovary at birth and following the weight of the other ovary. In adults, unilateral ovariectomy reduces the circulating level of ovarian steroids, so the feedback inhibition of pituitary secretion is reduced, FSH and LH secretion increases, and there is compensatory hypertrophy of the remaining ovary. As shown in Fig. 19, significant compensatory hypertrophy does not appear in young rats until they are 20-25 days of age. This suggests that negative feedback first occurs at about this age.

CONCLUSIONS

The data I have presented above represent samples from many different aspects of current research on brain-endocrine interactions. Let me close by saying that the interrelations between the brain and endocrine system are complex, multiple, varied and fascinating. They include not only relations in the adult but developmental phenomena as well. Factors such as gland sensitivity must be considered and must be kept in mind by all those interested in modeling the endocrine system.

I hope we will have more meetings like this one. In the meantime, I believe I speak for most if not all of us when I say that the meeting has been a benefit to all concerned; it certainly has been to me.

REFERENCES

1. Cahill, G.F. Jr., Verbal communication during discussion period, this conference.

2. Cantu, R.C., B.L. Wise, A. Goldfein, K. Gullixson, N. Fischer and W.F. Ganong. Proc. Soc. Exp. Biol. and Med. 114:10, 1963.

3. Cantu, R.C., G.G. Nahas and W.M. Manger. Proc. Soc. Exp. Biol. and Med. 122:434, 1966.

4. Crone, G. Acta Physiol. Scand. 59, Suppl. 213:29, 1963.

5. Etkin, W. Science 139:810, 1963

6. See Ganong, W.F., in A. Nalvandov, ed. Advances in Neuroendocrinology, Univ. of Ill. Press, Urbana, 1963.

7. Ganong, W.F., E.G. Biglieri and P.J. Mulrow, Recent Progress in Hormone Research 22:381, 1966.

8. Ganong, W.F. Review of Medical Physiology, 3rd Ed. Lange Medical Publications, Los Altos, Calif., 1967.

9. Ganong, W.F. and C.L. Kragt, in H.H. Cole and P.T. Cupps, eds., Reproduction in Domestic Animals,2nd Ed. Academic Press, N.Y. In press, 1968.

10. Gorski, R.A., Verbal communication during discussion period, this conference

11. Grodsky, G.M. and P.H. Forsham. Ann. Rev. Physiol. 28:347, 1966.

12. Harris, G.W. and D. Jacobsohn. Proc. Roy. Soc. B139:263, 1952.

BRAIN-ENDOCRINE INTERRELATIONS

13. Kragt, C.L., J. Dahlgren and W.F. Ganong. Third International Congress of Endocrinology Abstracts. In press, 1968.

14. Kragt, C.F. and W.F. Ganong, Endocrinology. In press, 1968.

15. Liddle, G.W., pp. 1-19, this volume.

16. Martini, L. and W.F. Ganong, eds. Neuroendocrinology, Academic Press, N.Y. Vol. I, 1966, Vol. II, 1967.

17. McCann, S.M., et. al. pp. 193-228, this volume.

18. Otsuka, K., T.A. Assaykeen, W.F. Ganong and W.H. Tu. Proc. Soc. Exp. Biol. and Med. 127:704, 1968.

19. Perkoff, G.T., K. Eik-Nes, C.A. Nugent, H.L. Fred, R.A. Nimer, L. Rush, L.T. Samuels and F.H. Tyler. J. Clin. Endocrinol. and Metab. 12:432, 1959.

20. Sherwood, L.M. New England J. Med. 278:663, 1968.

21. Williams, R.H., in R.H. Williams, ed., Textbook of Endocrinology, 4th ed. Saunders, Philadelphia, 1968.

22. Yates, F.E., Verbal communication during discussion period, this conference.

WILLIAM F. GANONG

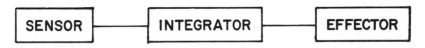

FIG. 1.   Organization of the nervous system.

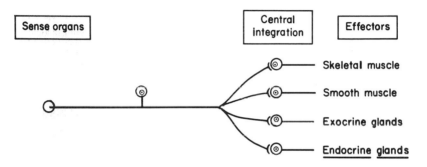

FIG. 2.   Effector mechanisms available to the nervous system.   From Ganong, W.F. in [16], reproduced with permission.

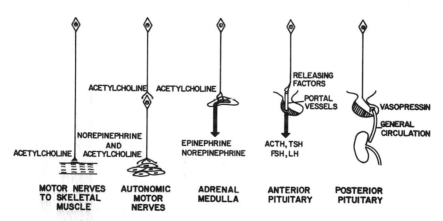

FIG. 3.   Diagrammatic representation of five situations in which humoral substances are released by neurons.   From [8], reproduced with permission.

BRAIN-ENDOCRINE INTERRELATIONS

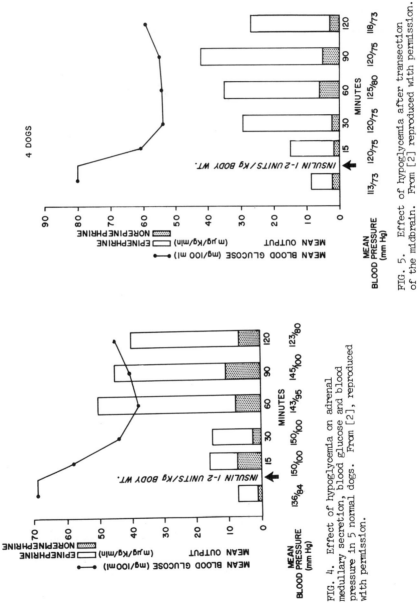

FIG. 5. Effect of hypoglycemia after transection of the midbrain. From [2] reproduced with permission.

FIG. 4. Effect of hypoglycemia on adrenal medullary secretion, blood glucose and blood pressure in 5 normal dogs. From [2], reproduced with permission.

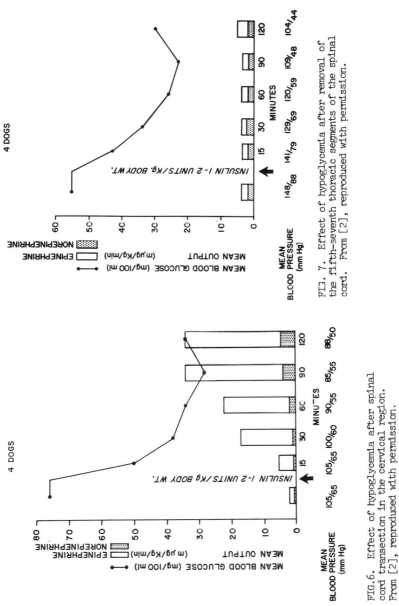

FIG. 7. Effect of hypoglycemia after removal of the fifth-seventh thoracic segments of the spinal cord. From [2], reproduced with permission.

FIG. 6. Effect of hypoglycemia after spinal cord transection in the cervical region. From [2], reproduced with permission.

BRAIN–ENDOCRINE INTERRELATIONS

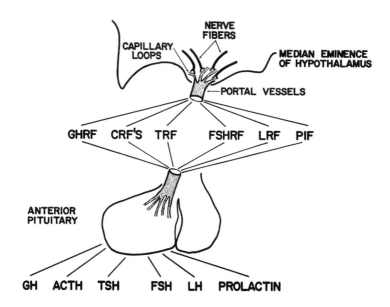

FIG. 8.   Diagrammatic summary of the neurovascular control mechanism
regulating anterior pituitary secretion. Control is exerted by
releasing factors and PIF secreted from nerve endings in the
hypothalamus into the blood stream and carried via the portal vessels
to the anterior pituitary. From [9], reproduced with permission.

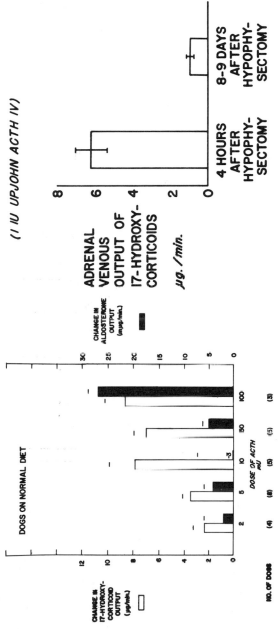

FIG. 9. Loss of ACTH responsiveness after hypophysectomy. Values are mean outputs in the adrenal vein after injection of one I.U. of ACTH. Vertical bars represent standard errors. From [8], reproduced with permission.

FIG. 10. Adrenal cortical responses to various doses of ACTH in hypophysectomized nephrectomized dogs fed a normal diet. The line above each column represents 1 standard error. From [7], reproduced with permission.

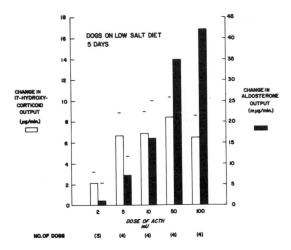

FIG. 11.   Effect of ACTH on adrenal cortical secretion
in dogs hypophysectomized and nephrectomized after being fed a low sodium diet for five days. From [7],
reproduced with permission.

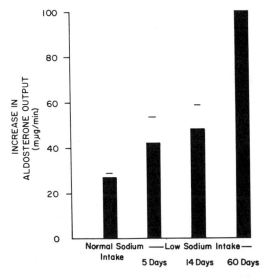

FIG. 12.   Increment in aldosterone secretion produced
by 100 mU of ACTH in dogs fed a normal diet and dogs
fed a low sodium diet for 5, 14 and 60 days.

LOW SODIUM DIET		
Sensitivity of secretory mechanism for:	Response to Angiotensin II	ACTH
ALDOSTERONE	+	+
17-HYDROXYCORTICOIDS	O	O

FIG. 13. Summary of effects of a low sodium diet on adrenal sensitivity.

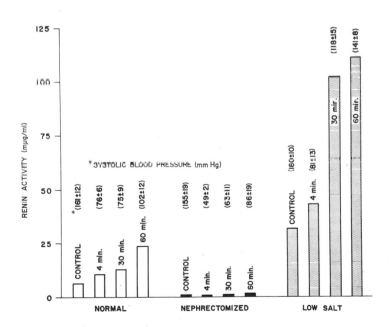

FIG. 14. Effect of hemorrhage on plasma renin levels in normal and nephrectomized dogs and in dogs fed a low sodium diet for 14 days. Data from [18].

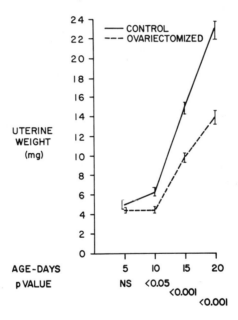

FIG. 15.   Effect of ovariectomy at birth
on uterine weight in rats. The vertical
lines represent the standard errors of
each mean.

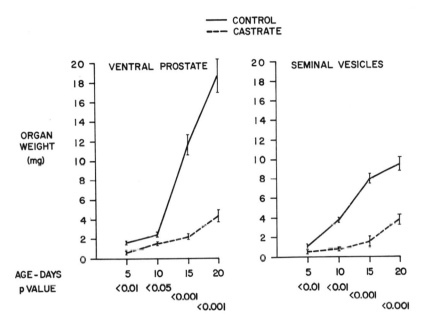

FIG. 16.   Effect of castration at birth on weight of sexual accessory organs in male rats.

BRAIN-ENDOCRINE INTERRELATIONS

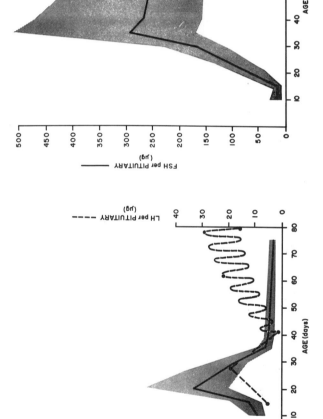

FIG. 17. Gonadotropin content of the pituitary of female rats at various ages. The solid line represents the mean FSH content and the shaded area represents the 95% confidence limits of the assays. The dash line represents the LH content, extrapolated from individual values (dots) in the literature. From [9], reproduced with permission.

FIG. 18. FSH content of the pituitary of male rats at various ages. From [9], reproduced with permission.

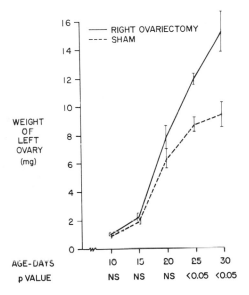

FIG. 19.   Compensatory ovarian hypertrophy in rats
at various ages following unilateral ovariectomy
at birth.

10. CONTROL SYSTEMS AND REGULATORY MECHANISMS OF THE BASIC

CELLULAR PROCESSES INVOLVING DNA AND RELATED MOLECULES

RENATO DULBECCO
The Salk Institute for Biological Studies

INTRODUCTION

In this paper I will adopt the point of view that the reader is primarily interested in the interactions and control mechanisms between biological elements, which are cells, considering them as black boxes and fundamentally ignoring how they work. By way of contrast and to complement the readers viewpoint I will look at the black box, the cell, and what is within it. Of course, it is a very complex subject as I am sure you are all aware. Some drastic simplification is therefore in order. Since the audience is mixed, of endocrinologists and engineers, I will mainly address myself to the engineers and make the simplification accordingly. The endocrinologists will hear things that may seem rather elementary because they hear them all the time, but they will forgive me, I hope.

A cell of a higher organism contains two compartments, the nucleus and the cytoplasm. There are membranes around each compartment, the nuclear and the plasma membrane; the nuclear membrane has holes that allow direct communication between the two compartments. The two membranes are in turn connected by other membranes. Thus the cell membranes are all connected into a unique system which may be important in the transmission of signals from the outside of the cells to the nucleus. A cell has two basic control systems. One is a control system for growth and multiplication; the other is for function. These two regulation systems may be somehow inter-related.

REGULATION OF SYNTHESIS OF CELLULAR CONSTITUENTS

A cell operates according to the following scheme. There is a repository of information, the DNA molecules, which are sequences of nucleotides many centimeters long. The four types of nucleotides alternate in a seemingly random way but this is a superfical impression because the sequence contains, in coded form, very precise messages. Every group of three bases corresponds to an informational unit, a triplet, of which there are billions. The DNA molecules are able to replicate to make more DNA. DNA can transfer its information to molecules of a different kind, RNA, which are similar to DNA because they are also made up of a nucleotide sequence. There is a main difference, however, because RNA is in smaller molecules. One can think of the DNA as being a dictionary of words, linearly encoded one after the other on a long string. The RNA in contrast reproduces one word or a small group of words at a time, in a separate molecule. A word is called a gene. The RNA, in turn, will transfer its information to protein molecules, which are the basic functional constituents of the cell. Some proteins make the structure of the cells, including membranes of which they are a fundamental constituent. Other proteins have a catalytic activity; they are the enzymes, and thus manufacture the vast number of substances present in the cell.

Regulation occurs through interactions between the various cell constituents. There are many known types of interactions and, of course, there must be many that are not now known. We can look at some important known types of interactions. Let's begin with the DNA molecules, which are long double helixes of two polynucleotide chains each formed by a backbone of alternating phosphate-ribose residues. Each sugar is connected to a base. All the bases point inward forming bonds between the two chains. There are two types of chemical groups that can be involved in interactions with other molecules. Groups of one type are the series of negative charges which lie on the outside of the molecules and are due to the presence of a phosphate residue in the backbone of each strand; then there are the bases themselves. One type of interaction characteristic of the bases is with certain planar molecules; since each pair of nucleotides (each attached to a different backbone) is planar, planar molecules such as acridines can become intercalated between them. It has been suggested that some steroid hormones may act in the same way because they have a planar configuration and appear to fit between two adjacent nucleotides. The outside of the DNA molecule, due to its negative charges, may interact with positively charged molecules of different kinds. Among these basic molecules are histones, which may be important in regulatory phenomena affecting the DNA.

Nucleic acids can interact also with large protein molecules. The interaction of protein with the nucleic acids can be specific, as can be recognized in many ways. First of all there are enzymes involved in DNA replication, which recognize the DNA, and probably certain specific parts of it. DNA replication begins at certain points and proceeds from then on; the replicating enzyme, therefore, recognizes the initiation points. It is not clear how this recognition occurs. It is likely that at the

REGULATION OF CELLULAR PROCESSES

recognition sites the DNA has a more complex structure than a simple double helix;
perhaps there are single-stranded loops, which would afford a large area of specificity through the exposed bases. Other enzymes are involved in the synthesis of the
RNA on DNA and they may also recognize specific sites of DNA in a similar way. A
group of enzymes are involved in the step in which information is transfered from RNA
to protein. This transfer occurs through special RNA molecules which each recognize
both a specific nucleotide triplet, and a certain amino acid. These RNA molecules,
called transfer RNAs, are small and have a peculiar structure, basically double stran-
ded but with single-stranded loops, and an overall flower-type shape. The amino acid
is attached at one end; at the other end, one of the loops contains a triplet which
is complementary to, and therefore can bind with, the triplet present in the RNA. The
whole act of information transfer from RNA to protein occurs on a large structure
called the ribosome. In order to connect the amino acid to its transfer RNA, an enzyme is needed, which must recognize a given transfer RNA among many others. Presumably this occurs through the interaction of a single-stranded loop of the RNA and
the enzyme.

Some kind of basic rule appears to emerge from these facts. Transfer of information between nucleic acids only involves a small number of elements: three nucleotides. In contrast, transfer of information between nculeic acids and protein
requires a much larger surface of interaction, obviously because of the different
way the information is stored in these molecules. Some evidence supporting this
statement will be given later on.

Among the protein molecules that interact with DNA, there is an important class,
whose function is regulation. These molecules are called repressors. A repressor
molecule recognizes a certain DNA sequence located at the beginning of the gene. This
property allows us to give a new and more complete definition of a gene. A gene is
a segment of DNA which begins with a special nucleotide sequence recognized by the
RNA-synthesizing enzyme and by a repressor (although it is not certain that there is
a repressor for each gene). The gene ends where another gene begins, always on the
same DNA chain. The end of a gene is also characterized by a characteristic sequence.
This explains how RNA molecules can be bonded to individual genes, whereas the genes
are connected in the DNA. The initiation point of a gene is essential for the synthesis of RNA; this is the regular phenomenon when the gene starts sending out his
information. Repressor molecules prevent this step, by recognizing and binding to
the initiation point. Presumably the initiation of RNA synthesis involves a much
smaller specificity than the binding of the repressor, since repressors are gene-
specific whereas RNA-synthesizing enzymes are not, to a large extent. The repressors are one of the basic tools for regulation of gene expression in cells.

What I have said so far has to do with one general mechanism of regulation, regulation of synthesis which can be summarized as follows. There is regulation of the
synthesis of DNA on DNA, and of RNA on DNA; it is likely that there are also mechanisms that regulate the synthesis of protein on RNA, although they are not known. The
effect of regulation at any level is to prevent the end results of the action of the
affected gene; ultimately, the protein specified by the gene is not made, and the cells
will be deficient for that particular function.

REGULATION OF FUNCTION OF CELLULAR CONSTITUENTS

I wish now to turn to a completely different type of regulation that occurs at the
level of the proteins after they have been synthesized and has to do with the function
of the proteins. This is an important regulatory mechanism in bacteria and perhaps
also in higher organisms. However, the latter statement is more an inference than a
conclusion based on facts. The regulation of function is based on a fundamental property of protein molecules, which has been understood during the last few years. This
is the ability of proteins to undergo characteristic structural changes from one shape
to another, called allosteric transitions. These transitions are possible owing to
the structure of protein molecules. They are very large molecules (molecular weight
up to a million or so), and usually are made up of subunits, which can be all equal
or of different kinds. Proteins with a very pronounced regulation based on allosteric
transition are usually made up of more than one type of subunit. A common situation
is to find two types of subunit. Each subunit is already a fairly large molecule,
containing several hundred amino acids in a long polypeptide chain; the chain is then
folded in many complex ways and kept in the folded state by intramolecular bonds con-
necting the various loops. These bonds are usually of low energy (e.g., hydrogen
bonds); they can suffer small degrees of distortion without requiring too much energy.
Thus the structure of a subunit can be changed from its regular configuration to a
somewhat different one simply by allowing a certain small amount of change (in length
or direction) in each of the constituent bonds. The energy barrier between the two
configurations is low and therefore is readily activated by heat at physiological temperature.

A common situation is that a protein with allosteric capabilities interacts with
two types of substances. One of these substances is the substrate, i.e., the substance on which the protein acts. We recognize that the protein is an enzyme because
it acts on a particular substrate. For instance, if it is proteolytic enzyme, it will
split peptide bonds, and the substrate will be a certain type of peptide bond. The
other substance recognized by the allosteric protein is the regulator. Regulatory

REGULATION OF CELLULAR PROCESSES

molecules can be quite different from the substrate. For instance, an extensively studied enzyme with allosteric properties, aspartic acid transcarbamylase, recognizes aspartic acid, an amino acid with two carboxyl groups, as its substrate. The regulatory molecule is cytidine triphosphate, a substance chemically unrelated to the substrate itself. However, cytidine triphosphate is a distant product of the reaction catalized by the enzyme. This gives a rationale for the regulation.

How do the allosteric changes happen? What seems to be quite clear on the basis of lots of work done over several years is that in the aspartic acid transcarbamylase the two types of subunits have different functions. One type of subunit has the enzymatic function and recognizes the substrate. The other type of subunit has regulatory function and recognizes the cytidine triphosphate. There are two subunits of each type in the same molecule. The mechanism of allosteric transition can be summarized as follows. The attachment of the regulatory molecule, as well as of the substrate, involves weak bonds so that there is a certain equilibrium between attached and free molecules. At a certain concentration of these molecules, the protein is associated with them for a certain proportion of the time. When the time is sufficiently long at a sufficiently high concentration of the molecules, a change in the structure of the enzyme is likely to occur. A regulatory subunit connected with a regulatory molecule changes configuration to one more energetically favorable; this causes a change of structure of the whole protein molecule, which affects its rate of interaction with the substrate. The total shape change of the transcarbamylase in the presence or absence of cytidine triphosphate is so large that it affects its sedimentation rate. When the regulatory molecule is removed, the enzyme returns to its original shape.

Now the end-results of these changes in the rate of the enzymatic reaction can be of various types. A common event is that the regulatory molecule causes a certain inhibition of the enzymic reaction at low concentrations of the substrate. This cooperative-type kinetics reveals the participation of more than one subunit in the process. Furthermore the dependence of the reaction rate on substrate concentration instead of being linear, as it is for enzymes without regulatory subunits, becomes s-shaped. In some cases the change of the shape of the curve is physiologically important. An example is hemoglobin, which has four subunits, and has an s-shaped dependence of bound oxygen on oxygen concentration. The changes in amount of bound oxygen corresponding to physiological changes in oxygen concentration are much larger than would be possible if the enzyme were just made up of one subunit and the curve were linear.

RENATO DULBECCO

REGULATION INVOLVING CELL MEMBRANES

It seems that other important aspects of regulatory phenomena involving the whole cell are centered around the plasma membranes, which may be an important regulatory element. A membrane is made up of a very large number of subunits connected to each other by weak bonds. The subunits contain protein and in addition lipids, which have fewer intramolecular bonds and thus increase the plasticity of the whole structure. Presumably the membrane subunits can undergo configuration shifts even more easily than proteins. It is most likely that within a given membrane there are many different types of subunits, each able to interact with a different type of regulatory molecule. The effect of interaction of molecules, or ions, outside or inside the cell, with the plasma membrane is especially dramatic in the case of the nerve cells. It is clear that the plasma membrane is an allosteric system built up of an almost infinite number of subunits. This is shown both by the observations of nerve cell membranes, and by theoretical calculations. The cooperative action of such a large number of subunits causes very sharp transitions from one configuration to another. Thus the dependence of bound ions to ion concentration assumes a very sharp s-shape, very close to a step function. As a consequence a membrane can be a true switching element as in the case of nerve cells.

SOME SPECIFIC ASPECTS AND EXAMPLES OF CONTROL AND REGULATION OF CELLULAR PROCESSES

I have so far described the basic elements of regulatory systems. Now we can ask some concrete questions about them. What do we specifically know about regulatory molecules? For instance, we have talked about repressors. Why do we say that there are repressors? Do we know any repressor? To answer these and similar questions we must turn to a much simpler system than a whole cell, because a cell is of such a complexity that it is a tremendous task to try to understand what happens to any one of its genes or of its proteins. Simplified systems usually involve viruses that contain DNA. The DNA of a virus has a much smaller number of genes than that of a cell; it is possible therefore to analyze the function of a gene of a virus with much greater ease than for a cellular gene. A useful subject for studying a gene repressor is a virus of bacteria called lambda. Whereas the DNA of the bacterium is about 1.2 mm long, that of the virus is approximately 15 microns, so there is a change of order of magnitude in the degree of complexity between bacterium and virus. When the virus is introduced into the cell, its DNA may become part of the cellular DNA; if this happens, it operates in the cell just as if it were a segment of the cellular DNA. Since the operation of the viral DNA is similar to that of the cel-

REGULATION OF CELLULAR PROCESSES

lular DNA, it can be used efficiently as a probe to see how the genes of the cell
themselves work.

The genes of this virus can be distinguished in three groups which will be called
the left group, the right group and the center group. These groups can be recognized
because the viral DNA molecules can be split in the middle by shearing, and then the
right and left parts can be separated by proper procedures, owing to slight differences in average base composition. It turns out that these three groups of genes are
physiologically very different from each other, as we can see by briefly examining
the biology of the virus. The virus is a small tadpole-like structure which attaches
to the cell surface and injects into it its DNA. The injected DNA within the cell has
two choices. One is to become inserted linearly in the cellular DNA. The other is
to start reproduction; then many new copies of the DNA are made and finally the cell
is lysed. When the virus reproduces itself, there are two stages in the process. In
the first stage the right genes are activated, and produce enzymes required for the
multiplication of the viral DNA. At this time the left genes don't work, so there is
a regulatory mechanism which recognizes only one group of genes. DNA replication occurs after the proper enzymatic machinery has been built by the function of the right
genes. DNA replication starts the function of the left genes, which then produce all
the protein molecules of the viral envelope, as well as an enzyme which conveniently
lyses the cell so the progeny virus can get out. When the other event, i.e. the in-
sertion of the viral DNA in the cellular DNA takes place, neither the right nor the
left genes operate, but only the center genes. As long as the association between
viral and cellular DNA persists, some of the center genes will be operating, but the
others will remain silent.

The problem now arises; why don't most genes work in the integrated viral DNA?
The answer is that one of the center genes produces a reprocessor, which acts on another gene of the center group, called the N gene. (The letter refers to some arbitrary ordering.) The N gene in turn once activated will make a product (so far
unknown), which is required for the activity of the right genes. We can think that
the product of the N genes recognizes some initiation point in the right segment of
the viral DNA, and by interacting with it, it will allow the synthesis of the RNA
corresponding to the right genes. Once this RNA is made, the corresponding proteins
will be synthesized as well. Among the right genes there is a gene designated as Q,
which makes a product required for the activity of the left genes. Thus the activation of the whole sets of genes involves a cascade phenomenon.

This complex mechanism has been unraveled by studying mutants of the viral DNA.
In a mutant one of the bases of a DNA triplet is changed, and therefore the protein
made by the mutated gene is different from the regular protein, and is usually non-

functional. Whenever the viral DNA has a mutation that makes one of the proteins non-functional, the cascade process is stopped at that step. By looking at the consequence of many different mutations in different genes the whole process has been reconstructed.

Of the substances involved in the cascade process only one is known, and it is the repressor specified by a gene of the center group. This repressor has been isolated out of the cell and purified to a considerable extent. It is a protein able to bind reversibly to the viral DNA as we postulated in our previous discussion. It is made up of subunits and its action is presumably controlled by allosteric change when it interacts with the DNA segment it recognizes.

Another known repressor regulates a bacterial gene which specifies the enzyme β-galactosidase. Thus repressors are not theoretical: they are available in the test tube.

Regulation by a repressor is negative, by preventing a specific synthesis. On the contrary the other two crucial genes of lambda, the N and the Q genes, apparently cause a positive regulation by producing a product that is required for a certain specific synthesis. A positive effect, however, could be obtained by a double negative mechanism, such as the production of an antirepressor that counteracts a repressor. There are examples in biology showing that what seems to be a positive action is actually a double negative. An example is the regulation of the β-galactosidase gene of bacteria. This gene is involved in the utilization of lactose, a disaccharide, which must be split by the β-galactosidase enzyme. If the cells are kept in the presence of lactose or other β-galactosides, lots of β-galactosidase is made in the cell; but if the β-galactoside is removed from the medium, soon the β-galactosidase will vanish from the cells. Thus the activity of the β-galactosidase gene is regulated. Historically, this was the first gene on which regulation was studied.

The genetic analysis of this system has shown that the β-galactosidase gene is regulated by the repressor that we already discussed. This repressor acts on a part of the β-galactosidase gene, the operator. When the repressor interacts with the operator, the RNA of the β-galactosidase gene (and of the other two genes of related function) is not made; consequently β-galactosidase is not made. When a β-galactoside is added to the medium, it seems to have a positive action, because it causes the enzymes to be made. In effect this is a double negative effect, because the β-galactoside inactivates the repressor, which is made all the time.

The study of repression of the β-galactosidase gene has also contributed much understanding about the nature of the interaction between regulatory molecules and their targets, which I mentioned at the beginning of this paper. Here we have a repressor that interacts with the DNA of a gene and prevents its transcription; natu-

REGULATION OF CELLULAR PROCESSES

rally attempts have been made to isolate mutants of the cell that would not recognize
the repressor. Such mutant cells should make the enzyme all the time, because they
should be insensitive to regulation by the repressor. In fact, such mutants were
found, but for a while it was surprising to find that they were all large structural
changes of the DNA, in which long sequences of nucleotides in the operator region were
missing. They were not point mutations affecting just one nucleotide of a triplet.
This result has led to the notion that the interaction between a protein molecule,
such as the repressor, and the DNA, requires a large surface of interaction. If there
is a change in just one nucleotide it will be essentially irrelevant for the interaction and will not be noticed. Only the deletion of a whole segment of DNA can prevent the interaction.

Author Index

AUTHOR INDEX

Numbers underlined designate those page numbers on which the complete literature citations are given.

AUTHOR INDEX

AUTHOR INDEX

Subject Index

SUBJECT INDEX

302